Praise for
The Busy Person's Guide to Permanent Weight Loss

"What makes this book so readable is its combination of good science and common sense, a rare combination in diet books. More importantly, it takes into account the compression of time in today's society, which compromises even the best dietary strategy."

—Barry Spears, Ph.D., Author, *The Zone*

"At last, a weight-loss guide for real people who live in the real world! As an M.D. with nutrition expertise, who sees patients every day who are seeking to lose weight, Dr. Jampolis gives readers what other diets don't: practical advice on healthier eating that they can follow no matter how busy their lives are."

—Anne M. Russell, Editor in Chief, *VIVmag*

"In *The Busy Person's Guide to Permanent Weight Loss*, Dr. Jampolis offers a realistic, lifestyle-based approach to weight loss that even the busiest person can accomplish. If lack of time has been your excuse for not losing weight and exercising regularly, this is the book for you!"

—Miriam Nelson, Ph.D., Author, *Strong Women Stay Young*

D0173492

THE BUSY PERSON'S
PERSON'S
GUIDE TO
PERMANENT
WEIGHT LOSS

MELINA B. JAMPOLIS, M.D.

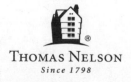

THOMAS NELSON
Since 1798

NASHVILLE   DALLAS   MEXICO CITY   RIO DE JANEIRO   BEIJING

Published in Nashville, Tennessee, by Thomas Nelson. Thomas Nelson is a registered trademark of Thomas Nelson, Inc.

Thomas Nelson, Inc., titles may be purchased in bulk for educational, business, fund-raising, or sales promotional use. For information, e-mail: SpecialMarkets@ThomasNelson.com

Calorie burn rate estimates are used courtesy of CyberSoft, Inc., makers of NutriBase Nutrition and Fitness Software, Phoenix, Arizona. All rights reserved.

The Busy Person's Guide to Permanent Weight Loss provides information of a general nature, and readers are strongly cautioned to consult with a physician or other healthcare professional before engaging in any of the programs described herein. This book is not to be used as an alternative method for conditions requiring the services of a personal physician.

Information contained in this book or in any other publication, article, Web site, etc. should not be considered a substitute for consultation with a board-certified doctor to address individual medical needs. Individual facts and circumstances will determine the treatment that is most appropriate. *The Busy Person's Guide to Permanent Weight Loss* Publisher and its Author, Melina Jampolis, M.D., disclaim any liability, loss, or damage that might result in the implementation of the contents of this book.

Formerly published as *The No Time to Lose Diet*.

Library of Congress Cataloging-in-Publication Data

Jampolis, Melina B.
    The busy person's guide to permanent weight loss / Melina B. Jampolis.
      p. cm.
    Includes bibliographical references.
    ISBN 978-0-7852-2218-7 (hardcover)
    ISBN 978-1-4016-0408-0 (repak)
  1. Reducing diets. 2. Weight loss. I. Title.
RM222.2.J357 2007
613.2'5—dc22

                        2006028516

Printed in the United States of America

08 09 10 11 12 RRD 7 6 5 4 3 2 1

To my Grandma Lillie, the light of my life,
and to my parents for raising me
to believe that anything is possible

CONTENTS

ACKNOWLEDGMENTS

I would like to acknowledge several people without whom this book would not have been possible:

First, Alex Marr, who encouraged me for years to write this book and was probably one of the few who had no doubts that I could and should do it;

Nancy Saslow of MegTV for "discovering" me and giving me the opportunity to disseminate my nutrition and diet message on a larger scale than I ever thought possible;

My agent, Shannon Miser-Marven, for her commitment to this project and her patience and understanding with a novice doctor-author;

My editors, Kristen Parrish and Paula Major, whose thoughtful comments and suggestions truly made this a better book;

Emily Scott Pottruck for those motivating brainstorming sessions over a healthy lunch;

My brilliant mother, Barbara, to whom I must give credit for the title of the book, which perfectly depicts my approach; and my sister, Ami, for her friendship and support;

And finally, thank you to all of my wonderful patients over the years, who have inspired me, believed in me, shared their successes and failures with me, and without whom I would never have had the insight and motivation to write this book. I wish them all a lifetime of health and happiness.

INTRODUCTION

I am a diet doctor. This statement may seem unusual in the diet-book world, since most popular diet-book authors begin their books with the disclaimer "I am *not* a diet doctor." Most of these best-selling authors are, instead, psychologists, personal trainers, celebrities, scientists, heart doctors, and sometimes just people who have been successful at losing weight. Almost none of these "experts" interact directly with real people struggling with weight loss on a daily basis. I do. I see patients trying to lose weight, all day, every day. I witness firsthand their weekly struggles and successes, and in the process I have learned a *lot* about successful weight loss.

I also hosted a TV show, FitTV's *Diet Doctor*, in which I evaluated ten of the most popular diets in the country. I met with the diet author or expert to discuss the diet in detail and then returned home and helped a local dieter get started on my own modified version of the diet. One of the most important things that I learned through both seeing patients and filming the TV show is that most diets fail because people simply do not have the time or energy to follow them for the long-term. They also lack the tools to incorporate them permanently in their lives. This book will solve both of these problems.

Whether you have a busy social life, a hectic travel schedule, a demanding job, a chaotic household, a new baby, no time for exercise, or limited time to cook or shop regularly, I have created a program that can and will work for you. Throughout this book, I have tried to address every challenging situation that my patients have faced over the years, and I have developed numerous strategies to successfully conquer them. Whether you need ideas for breakfast on the go, no-cook dinners, eating-out strategies, travel-eating tips, or ways to maximize your exercise in the least amount of time, you will find everything you need to successfully and permanently lose weight in the most time-efficient way possible.

> Whether you have a busy social life, a hectic travel schedule, a demanding job, a chaotic household, a new baby, no time for exercise, or limited time to cook or shop regularly, I have created a program that can and will work for you.

In addition to being time efficient, this book addresses all aspects of weight loss, not just nutrition. Again, through working with patients on an everyday basis, I have learned that, to be successful, it is critical to address the behavior and exercise components of weight loss *in addition* to the nutrition component. Since most people do not have time to go to the gym for an hour five times per week, and most cannot afford the time or expense of seeing a therapist to work through their eating issues, I have come up with proven exercise and behavior strategies to help you build the solid foundation necessary for permanent weight loss.

Another rather unique element of this book is that I have personalized it based on your individual needs. A second common reason that most diets fail is that there is no "one size fits all" when it comes to weight loss. Many factors determine what diet will work best for you, including genetics, medical history, activity level, age, sex, and even your food preferences. To be successful in the long-term, a weight-loss program must take these factors into consideration. Since I cannot see you in my office and customize your program myself, I developed the Carbohydrate Calculator to help you figure out what level of starchy carbohydrates is most appropriate for you. In addition, rather than providing precise recommendations for other food groups, I offer ranges of daily servings so that you have some flexibility each day to eat the foods you really enjoy.

As a physician, I make it a top priority to stay very current on the latest research in the field of obesity. I attend medical meetings and read both nutrition and obesity medical journals on a regular basis. Keeping up with the rapidly expanding field of obesity research while working with patients day after day allows me to quickly translate the latest weight-loss advances into practical approaches for my patients. Hence, I have combined the most important nutritional concepts both for weight loss and optimal health. Some suggestions may be familiar; others may not.

While some nutrition experts may argue with certain aspects of my approach, my goal throughout this book is to mix the best scientific evidence with a practical and real-

life approach. I do not expect perfection. If I could not follow a specific recommendation all of the time, then I do not
expect you to either. You will not always eat perfectly while
following this program. My goal is simply for you to make
healthier choices most of the time.

Finally, one the best features of this book is that it is filled
with examples from actual patients. The case studies you
will read are about real people just like you—people with
busy schedules, stressful lives, and very little time or energy
to dedicate to weight loss. They represent a very diverse
group of individuals, with equally diverse eating, exercise,
and behavioral issues. Yet each was able to take my general
principles, meal ideas, and shopping lists and figure out a
weight-loss approach that was just right. I hope that you will
not only be inspired by their successes, but that you may
learn from their mistakes and also realize that *you* can make
mistakes and still achieve long-term success.

Please view this book as a permanent weight-loss resource
and guide rather than as a short-term, quick-fix diet. Do not
feel that you have to follow every suggestion or make every
change I recommend. Some of the strategies may work well for
you; others may not be relevant. Your job is to use the information and concepts presented in this book to find the right
approach for you, and then try to stick with this approach
most—but not necessarily all—of the time.

At this point, I hope you are convinced that this weight-
loss book *is* different and *can* work for you, even with your
busy life. So let's get started.

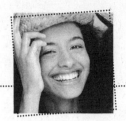

ONE

The Busy Person's Basic Principles

WL is a sixty-eight-year-old man who came to see me last year at his doctor's recommendation. He needed to lose weight, had significant heart disease, and had just undergone angioplasty in January. He also had issues with chronic pain, which severely limited his ability to exercise, and he felt that his new pain medications had caused him to gain forty pounds. He had "been on every diet on the face of the planet," and he was very skeptical that I would be able to help him lose weight permanently. He explained that he lived alone and did not cook at all. In fact, he used the inside of his oven to store papers. He was very clear that if my program required cooking, it would not work for him. He also defiantly told me that he loved cookies and often ate entire bags in one sitting. He laughed when I asked him about his daily exercise regimen, insisting that his pain made even walking for more than ten minutes virtually impossible.

I remember listening to WL that first day and thinking that I was just not going to get through to him; he was simply too set in his ways. I actually told him that I was not sure I could help him as I wasn't certain that he was open to being helped. We even discussed his signing up for only one visit instead of a full program and if he did not perceive value in my suggestions that we part ways. I did not want to battle him weekly for the next six months.

He agreed to follow the program, and we began working together the next week. WL preferred simplicity in his eating plan, which I find to be the case with most men. The first week he cut his eating dramatically and lost four pounds eating mostly protein, vegetables, and protein bars. He felt great, but I did not want him losing weight so quickly, as I wanted to preserve his muscle mass as much as possible, especially with his limited exercise ability. I insisted that he add at least one serving of fruit, replace one of his daily protein bars with yogurt as a snack, and add beans to his salad to increase his fiber intake and slow his weight loss a bit. He continued losing weight steadily, averaging about two and a half pounds per week. After one month, he hit a plateau and did not lose weight for two weeks. This is very common among dieters, and I find the first plateau to be a critical time because most people give up in frustration if they feel they are working hard to lose weight, but the scale is not responding.

At this point WL surprised me. While he was disappointed, rather than becoming frustrated and giving up, he decided to add exercise to the equation. I told him that I thought resistance bands might be easier on his joints. He could do a few exercises when he felt up to it, and quit if it became too painful. I also encouraged him to aim for five- to ten-minute walking bouts whenever he felt able. He came back the next week with a three-pound weight loss and reported walking four times and exercising his upper body with the resistance bands fifteen minutes a day. He was happy about the weight loss but decided that he was bored with breakfast and wanted a change. I recommended that he alternate his usual protein-bar breakfast with a whole wheat English muffin and peanut butter.

Every week WL would come in with restaurant take-out menus and grocery-store flyers and we would find one or two healthy options to add to his diet to prevent boredom. Six weeks later, WL hit another weight-loss plateau after one of his doctors started him on a new pain medication. This time, he was not disappointed at all. He told me that he knew he was on the right track, he was happy with what he was eating, and he was confident that he would begin losing weight again when the medication issue was sorted out. The next week, down twenty-eight pounds at this point, he got some great news from his doctor: his triglycerides had dropped 30 points (a 21-percent reduction), his bad cholesterol had dropped 23 points (a 31-percent reduction), and his good cholesterol had increased an incredible 27 points (a 61-percent increase).

Inspired by his success both in weight loss and general health, WL sailed through Thanksgiving and Christmas with ease, treating himself to small portions of anything he felt like, including a Christmas cookie or two every now and then, but filling up with the healthier options, like turkey and vegetables.

I'm happy to say that six months after that initial consultation, during which I never in a million years would have guessed that WL would be one of my most rewarding successes, he is down fifty-four pounds and is now at 18 percent body fat. He will be celebrating his seventieth birthday next year in the best shape of his life. He calls me his *miracle worker*, but the reality is that he was ready to lose weight for good this time and was completely committed to making a permanent lifestyle change. I simply gave him the tools to succeed and a healthy dose of moral support along the way.

● ● ●

Now that you have a bit of inspiration, let's get started with The Busy Person's principles that were so successful for WL. These principles address the three basic components of successful weight loss: nutrition, exercise, and behavior. It is important to remember that these principles are not rules set in stone, but rather guidelines upon which you will build your own unique weight-loss program. I describe them to my patients as the infrastructure, or foundation, of a successful, realistic, time-efficient, long-term weight-loss program.

> If you ate a higher percentage of protein at most meals and snacks, that alone could burn up to 100 extra calories per day, which could help you lose twelve pounds per year.

THE BUSY PERSON'S PRINCIPLE 1: TRY TO EAT
SOME FORM OF PROTEIN WITH EVERY MEAL AND SNACK

Eating protein with every meal and snack is one of the keys to successful weight loss and maintenance, for three important reasons: the metabolic effects of protein, blood sugar stabilization, and hunger control. I will explain all three in detail below, and you will notice that I refer back to these points throughout the book.

Maximizing Metabolism with Protein

Let's start with the metabolic effects of eating protein. The direct advantage is due to a small but important component of your metabolism, called the *thermic effect* of food, which is the amount of calories used in the digestion and absorption of food. The thermic effect of food makes up about 10 percent of your daily calorie requirements. The higher the thermic effect of a particular food, the more calories you burn simply processing that food. Protein has the highest thermic effect, followed by carbohydrates and then fat.

One study showed that the thermic effect of a higher-protein meal was approximately double the thermic effect of a high-carbohydrate meal.[1] While overall this effect is relatively small and its importance in dieting widely debated, even a modest increase in the number of calories burned can have significant effects, both short-term and long-term, on weight loss.

Another research study found that people burned an additional twenty-five calories after consuming a high- versus low-protein drink.[2] This may not seem like much on its own, but if you ate a higher percentage of protein at most meals and snacks, that alone could burn up to 100 extra calories per day, which could help you lose twelve pounds per year. In addition, it could also help offset the 5- to 10-percent drop in metabolism that often accompanies dieting.

More on the Metabolic Advantage of Protein

Fat is the body's most efficient fuel. Your body does not utilize a lot of energy (calories) to turn the fat you eat into the fat you use or store in your body. While carbohydrates have less than half the calories per gram of fat, they, too, are relatively efficient fuel sources and require a fairly small amount of energy to be converted into a form your body can use.

Protein, on the other hand, is not as efficiently used by the body. Significantly more energy is required for the breakdown and rebuilding of proteins and for the conversion of protein to carbohydrates. Therefore, a higher-protein diet has a greater calorie cost. While this effect is not large and depends on everything you eat, not just the amount of protein, it can add up to a metabolic advantage for weight loss.

But before you speed off to your local butcher, this does *not* mean that you should consume huge amounts of protein at each meal to get an even bigger boost to your metabolism. This *will not* work. Eating more calories than you need at *any* meal will far outweigh the modest increase in calories burned eating protein.

Maximizing Metabolism Through Muscle Mass

You have probably noticed that when you diet, you don't just lose fat—you lose muscle mass, water, and even a small amount of bone mass. It's just one of the harsh realities of weight loss.

You may think this is not a problem, since the scale is dropping, but one pound of muscle burns approximately thirty-five to fifty calories per day, while fat burns very little. So when you lose muscle, you *lower* your metabolism. Again, this may not seem like a lot of calories, but it can add up over time and is one possible explanation for weight-loss plateaus and weight regain during maintenance. The most effective way of preventing muscle loss and maintaining your metabolism is by using your muscles in weight training or exercise and by not losing weight too quickly. Research also shows that a higher-protein diet, especially when combined with exercise, is much better at preserving muscle mass.[3] This effect may be even more important as you age since protein is absorbed less efficiently and muscle is harder to build due to hormonal changes.

Hopefully, I have convinced you that moderately increasing your protein intake has significant metabolic advantages that play a primary role in weight loss. Here's more on metabolism:

MORE ON METABOLISM

What is *metabolism*? Metabolism is your body's total daily energy requirements. *Total metabolic rate* (TMR) is essentially made up of three components: *resting metabolic rate* (RMR); physical activity, including both exercise and general daily activity level; and calories required for digesting and absorbing food (also known as the *thermic effect* of food).

Resting metabolic rate (RMR). The rate at which you burn calories at rest, RMR is the minimum number of calories your body needs to keep you alive through breathing, brain and heart function, and more. RMR makes up 60 to 75 percent of your daily caloric requirements. RMR has a strong genetic component, but several things can affect it; some you can control, and others you can't. It is important to understand what you can control and do everything you can to maximize and maintain your TMR while losing weight.

Lean body mass (LBM) (muscle, bone, tissues, water). Greater LBM results in higher RMR. Since men generally have more muscle mass than women, their metabolism is usually 10 to 20 percent higher too. It is important for dieters, especially women, to try to increase lean body mass or, at the very least, minimize the loss of LBM by losing weight more slowly. This is the most variable component of RMR and, therefore, the area in which you have the most control.

Age. RMR decreases with age. This is due to natural changes in your body's physiology and its loss of muscle mass. Physical activity also decreases with aging, so you often get a double hit to your metabolism. Women, on average, lose about 3 percent of their LBM per decade. Research shows that it is never too late to build muscle, so it is critical to incorporate strength training into any permanent weight-loss program.[4]

Crash dieting or severe undereating decreases RMR. If you

drop your calories significantly below your basic requirements, your body will slow your metabolism 5 to 10 percent
within forty-eight hours. Your body may also be forced to use
muscle for energy, which can also lower your metabolism.

Hormones. During the second half of the menstrual cycle,
hormonal changes cause a slight increase in RMR, which is
why many women often feel hungrier during this time. It's
OK to eat a little more before your period.

Thyroid disease. An underactive thyroid (although not as
common as most would like) lowers RMR and is one reason
some women have difficulty losing weight. If you are struggling with weight loss, have your doctor make sure that your
thyroid function is normal.

Medications. This area is less understood by physicians, but
there are several medications that may affect metabolism.
Talk to your doctor about any medications you take that may
be affecting yours.

Physical activity level (PAL). PAL represents 15 to 25 percent
of your TMR and is the most variable component. It is also the
area where you have the most control day by day. In very
active people, PAL accounts for a larger portion of total metabolic rate. PAL includes more than just exercise. If you are
active at work—for example, a teacher who stands most of

the day—you will have a higher PAL than someone who sits at a computer all day. It is important to increase PAL as much as possible during weight loss and maintenance.

Thermic effect of food is approximately 10 percent of total metabolic rate, so the mere act of eating plays an important, albeit smaller, role.

The Importance of Blood Sugar Control in Weight Loss

The second reason for eating protein with each meal or snack is that protein stabilizes blood sugar. Why is this important for weight loss? Keeping blood sugar relatively stable helps you control hunger and cravings. Foods that are broken down quickly into simple sugars cause a rapid rise in blood sugar, followed by an equally rapid fall. Low blood sugar triggers hunger and lowers energy (and often mood) levels. This can lead to sugar and carbohydrate cravings since sugary foods raise blood sugar most quickly. You have probably experienced this effect after eating a high-sugar or high-carb breakfast, such as a bagel or donut and orange juice. Your energy likely peaked initially due to the large "sugar rush" but probably dropped just as quickly, leaving you counting the minutes until lunch or taking several trips to the coffee cart to keep you awake and alert.

Food Combining for Optimal Blood Sugar Control

While the type of carbs you eat is one of the most important factors for stabilizing blood sugar, the combination of foods can also play an important role. By combining a high-carbohydrate food that raises blood sugar quickly with a high-protein (or -fat) food that raises blood sugar much more slowly, your blood sugar will rise and fall more gradually, decreasing hunger and cravings. The low-carb diet craze focused on cutting carbohydrates as much as possible to stabilize blood sugar. This approach does work, but life without carbohydrates can be difficult to maintain and can leave you feeling tired and depressed. Eating some form of protein with every meal and snack is a much simpler and healthier way of achieving the same goal.

> The low-carb diet craze focused on cutting carbohydrates as much as possible to stabilize blood sugar. This approach does work, but life without carbohydrates can be difficult to maintain and can leave you feeling tired and depressed.

The Key to Hunger-Free Dieting

The final benefit of eating protein with most meals and snacks addresses a problem many dieters often face: hunger. Calorie for calorie, protein appears to be more filling than carbohydrates or fat. Research has shown that people living in the real world, not research labs, eat less and feel fuller when they eat a higher protein diet.[5] This effect may be especially significant with a higher-protein breakfast. The reason for this increased fullness with protein relates in part to the effect of protein on blood sugar but probably more importantly involves hormones in your gut and brain that trigger the sensation of fullness.

More Protein = Better Maintenance

Research shows that protein not only helps people losing weight to feel less hungry, but it also helps with weight maintenance. In one study, people who ate a higher percentage of protein during maintenance regained much less weight, and the weight that was regained was mainly muscle, not fat.[6] Don't forget that balance is important. Do not eat *only* protein—you need carbohydrates for your body to function optimally, and healthy fats to make many of the hormones essential for living and abundant health.

THE BUSY PERSON'S PRINCIPLE 2:
TRY TO EAT EVERY THREE TO FOUR HOURS

This principle is important for many of the same reasons as the first principle: to maintain lean body mass, to keep blood sugar stable, and to minimize hunger. While the thermic effect of eating more frequently is not significant, the effect of more frequent protein-based meals on maintaining muscle mass *is* significant. Research in both athletes and obese people shows that when given low-calorie diets, those who consumed their calories in five or six smaller meals a day—instead of two or three larger meals—lost less muscle mass.[7, 8, 9] Again, maintaining muscle is critical for minimizing the inevitable drop in your metabolism with weight loss and is even more important for preventing weight regain.

In addition, by having several smaller meals throughout the day rather than two or three large meals, your blood sugar level remains more stable because you are not taking in large quantities of food followed by long periods without food. Stabilized blood sugar keeps your energy more constant throughout the day and minimizes sugar cravings. Eating more frequently seems to be particularly important for women, who are genetically programmed to graze throughout the day rather than gorge.[10]

Finally, by not waiting more than three or four hours between meals or snacks, your hunger level is more manageable. This is important for successful weight loss from a behavioral standpoint, as it is much easier to make good meal and snack choices and to stop eating after an appropriate amount of food if you are not famished.

Imagine sitting down to dinner when you haven't eaten anything since lunch seven hours ago. If you are eating out, the first thing you will probably face is the bread or chip basket, the bowl of nuts at the bar, or the smell of french fries at the McDonald's drive-thru. At home, you may confront the leftover cookies from the party you had over the weekend, or your kid's macaroni and cheese. If you did not have an afternoon snack, your blood sugar is probably near an all-time low for the day. This signals your brain to get food and get it fast—no time to chop veggies or wait for your salad appetizer. And since it takes about twenty minutes for your brain to register fullness, you will probably be long past your fourth slice of bread, large fries, or halfway through the cookie plate by the time you are no longer "starving."

Don't make things more difficult or set yourself up for failure by putting yourself in this situation. Make sure that you eat a protein-containing meal or snack every three to four hours, especially in the afternoon. Try to eat before you get really hungry, but *never* force yourself to eat if you are not hungry just because four hours have passed. Everyone is different. If you don't get hungry between meals, skip the snacks. But if you arrive at meals ravenous, it is essential to have a snack in between. And if you aren't hungry in the afternoon but start feeling hungry on your way out to dinner, grab a little lean protein or a piece of fruit to take the edge off. It won't spoil your dinner, and it will allow you to make much better choices.

THE BUSY PERSON'S PRINCIPLE 3:
EAT THE RIGHT CARBOHYDRATES
IN THE RIGHT QUANTITY AT THE RIGHT TIME

Before I describe what I mean by the "right carbohydrates," I want to explain when, where, and why carbs went wrong. In the '80s and early '90s, fat was seen as the nutrition villain. As a result, a lot of the big food companies cut the fat in many of their products, including cookies, crackers, ice cream, and frozen dinners. Unfortunately, they had to replace the fat with something, and advances in food processing allowed inexpensive new sweeteners, like high-fructose corn syrup; refined sugar; and highly refined, processed carbohydrates to cheaply fill the gap. The problem is that the processing removes most of the vitamins, minerals, and fiber, leaving only rapidly digested, nutrient-depleted carbohydrates, salt, and— in many cases—dangerous fats.

In the past thirty years, these processed snacks, convenience foods, and soft drinks have become a staple in the American diet. Not only are many of them low-fat or nonfat, they are also cheap, fast, convenient, and tasty. With less and less time for home-cooked meals, consumption of these foods, along with fast food made from similar products, has grown exponentially. Unfortunately, the cost-savings benefits and ease made possible through modern food processing have a major downside: obesity.

Many nutritionists and obesity experts (including myself) believe that the tremendous increase in highly processed and/or sugary carbohydrates—including sugary snack foods, fast food, baked goods made with refined white flour, chips, and soft drinks—has contributed to the current obesity crisis in this country.

In the late '90s, with our nation's obesity and obesity-related diseases, like diabetes and heart disease, hitting record levels while we were supposedly following a low-fat, high-carbohydrate diet, attention turned to cutting carbohydrates instead of fat. Low-carb diets emerged into the public spotlight, and suddenly double bacon cheeseburgers without the bun were considered health food. You probably know dozens of people who lost weight initially on low-carb diets such as Atkins and South Beach. You may even have tried one yourself, vowing to banish bread, pasta, potatoes, fruit, and sweets for good. Perhaps you felt terrific and lost a lot of weight. More likely, however, you felt tired, deprived, bored, and constipated and began fantasizing about pizza or planning your visit to the local bakery the instant you reached your goal weight.

Low-carbohydrate diets can work well in the short-term for some, but most people have a hard time sticking to them for the long haul. A life without English muffins, sandwiches, chicken-noodle soup, apples, chocolate-chip cookies, or cereal can get very monotonous and can be challenging to maintain, particularly if you do not have a lot of time to shop and cook or if you have an active social life. In addition, omitting whole grains and fruit for extended periods undoubtedly has negative health consequences.

The Quantity of Carbohydrates Does Matter

Some obesity experts now believe it is not the quantity of carbohydrates that should be addressed for weight loss but rather the quality. Based on my experience working with thousands of patients trying to lose weight, I do not completely agree. There is no doubt that the quality of carbohydrates *is* very important, but I believe that the quantity is equally important and must be adjusted for each person. In my practice, I find that patients have very different levels of carbohydrate tolerance and sensitivity, and therefore it is critical to customize the amount for each person. In addition, I believe that the timing of carbohydrate intake is also important. I'll explain what I mean by the right carbohydrates at the right time here, and in the next chapter you will calculate exactly how many carbs you need for optimal weight loss.

When people talk about carbohydrates, they are usually referring to bread, pasta, and potatoes. But carbohydrates actually exist in lots of foods, including grains, fruits, vegetables, and dairy. All carbohydrates (except fiber—more on that later) are eventually broken down into basic sugars, your body's favorite source of fuel. So what makes some carb-containing foods better than others for weight loss? The quality *and* quantity of carbohydrates that they contain.

Let's talk about quality first. One of the best ways to evaluate carbohydrate quality in a particular food is to consider the effect of that food on blood-sugar levels, a value known as the *glycemic index*, or *GI*. Basically, the GI ranks foods according to how much a standard amount of a particular food raises blood sugar over a two-hour period. Most vegetables and dairy have a low glycemic index, while some fruits and many grains have a higher glycemic index. Why does the glycemic index of food matter? High GI foods are broken down very quickly into simple sugars. This often leads to an exaggerated release of insulin. One of insulin's most important jobs is to transfer sugar out of your blood into your fat, muscle, or liver. So basically, insulin feeds your fat cells—not a good thing if you are trying to lose weight!

While insulin is critical for survival (type 1 diabetics, who can't make insulin, would die without it), too much insulin promotes excess fat storage and prevents fat breakdown. Worse, too much insulin can cause fat accumulation around your waistline (the most dangerous kind for your heart), and higher levels may increase your risk of certain types of cancer. If you eat a high-glycemic diet on a regular basis for a long period of time, your body may become less sensitive to insulin or may simply not be able to keep up with the demand, leading to type 2 diabetes.

Glycemic Load and Weight Loss

Eating a lower-glycemic diet helps control hunger levels and may decrease your risk of heart disease and diabetes even without weight loss.[11] While some suggest that it may help in weight loss, I don't believe the glycemic index alone is that helpful. A more useful value is the *glycemic load* (GL), which takes into account the actual amount of carbohydrates in an average serving of a given food. By factoring in the quantity and the quality of carbohydrates per serving, you get a better idea of the impact on blood sugar and insulin. In the following box you will find the equation used for calculating the glycemic load. The significance is more easily understood through the examples shown there. These examples also clarify why carrots should not be off-limits for dieters as most low-carb-diet supporters might lead you to believe. If you are interested, you can learn a lot more about the glycemic index and glycemic load in *The New Glucose Revolution*.[12]

Glycemic Load = (Glycemic Index x
Carbohydrates per serving) / 100

GL less than or equal to 10 = Low

GL 11–19 = Medium

GL greater than or equal to 20 = High

Glycemic Index of carrots = 49
Carbohydrates per ½ cup serving (cooked) = 5 g.
Glycemic Load = (49 x 5) / 100 = 2.5

Glycemic Index of pretzels = 83
Carbohydrates per 1 ounce serving = 20 g.
Glycemic Load = (83 x 20) / 100 = 16

Glycemic Index of Corn Flakes cereal = 92
Carbohydrates per 1 cup serving = 26 g.
Glycemic Load = (92 x 26) / 100 = 24

Glycemic Index of instant white rice = 87
Carbohydrates per ¾ cup serving = 42 g.
Glycemic Load = (87 x 42) / 100 = 36

As you can see from these examples, the quantity of carbohydrates is just as important as the quality in determining the impact of a food on blood sugar. Note that neither value can be used alone for weight loss.

Don't get too caught up in the details of the glycemic index or glycemic load. Instead, think about the "big picture" and focus on eating mainly whole-grain, unprocessed carbohydrates with fewer added sugars, in controlled quantities. Since grains, sugars, and starchy carbohydrates are the most concentrated forms of carbohydrates and contribute the greatest number of calories to the typical American diet, simply cutting back on these foods can improve your diet significantly. Sugar alone makes up about 25 percent of the average American's daily caloric intake, so by simply reducing sugar (without replacing it with something else), you will more than likely lose weight and improve your health. Again, carbohydrate sensitivity varies, but it is important to adjust and monitor starchy carbohydrate intake closely, which is why I developed the Carbohydrate Calculator worksheet you will complete in the next chapter.

The Best Carbohydrate Sources for Weight Loss

Since most vegetables contain a very small number of carbohydrates but lots of fiber, vitamins, water, minerals, and phytonutrients, you can consume them in much larger quantities.

Fruit is also a very good source of fiber, vitamins, minerals, and phytonutrients, and therefore plays an important role in optimal health. But some fruits have a moderately high glycemic index and can affect blood sugar and weight loss when eaten alone or in large quantities. I recommend that higher-sugar fruits always be combined with a little protein or fat, and serving sizes should be monitored somewhat. Lower-sugar fruits can be consumed alone, and quantities are not as important, but fruit still has calories and should not be eaten in unlimited quantities.

The final source of carbohydrates is dairy, which contains *lactose*, also known as *milk sugar*. Dairy naturally combines carbohydrates with lean protein, so it has a low glycemic index and load. For optimal health and weight loss, avoid dairy products that have large amounts of added sugars or fats.

When to Eat Carbohydrates

Now that you understand more about the quality of carbohydrates, let's discuss the timing of your carb intake, especially grains and starchy carbohydrates. I like to tell my patients to think of grains and starchy carbs as fuel, since they are the most concentrated source of carbohydrates. When do you need fuel the least? Usually at night, when you are less active. For this reason, I strongly recommend limiting starchy carbohydrates at night. Research shows that eating larger meals at night is associated with obesity.[13] While no research study that I know of has looked at the timing of carbohydrate intake, I have found in my practice that limiting starchy carbs at night works incredibly well for my patients, for two reasons.

First, starchy carbohydrates are very easy to overeat. Do you frequently sit in front of the TV, popping steak cubes or cherry tomatoes into your mouth, instead of chips, crackers, or popcorn? Do you regularly devour two apples and a quart of yogurt after supper, instead of ice cream and cookies? And do you go out to dinner and fill up on shrimp cocktail and salad instead of bread and butter before your entrée arrives? My guess is that your answer is *no*. Since most people tend to overeat starchy—not healthy—carbohydrates later in the day, limiting starchy carbohydrates at night will help lower your daily (and nightly) caloric intake at the very time when you are also the least active. This combination can help maximize fat burning.

Second, limiting starchy carbohydrates at night helps address a major deficiency in the American diet: inadequate vegetable intake. If you are not eating starches at night, you are going to have to eat more vegetables to fill yourself up. It is amazing how much more creative and consistent my patients become with vegetable choices at night when they have fewer other options.

Regarding timing of carbohydrate intake, it is also important to balance carbohydrate intake throughout the day. If you eat two servings of bread at breakfast, you may want to save your fruit for a snack or lunch. If you have a large serving of fruit with lunch, cut back on the kidney beans on your salad. If you plan to eat pasta at night, skip the bread at lunch. While I prefer that you eat starchy carbohydrates— bread, cereal, pasta, and rice—at breakfast or lunch, it is most crucial to learn to balance your choices over the course of the day for optimum weight loss.

Here is a summary of the key carbohydrate points:

- Focus mainly on low-glycemic-load carbohydrates.
- Pay attention to quantities of starchy, processed, and sugary carbohydrates.
- Evenly spread carbohydrates throughout the day.
- Limit grains, starches, and sugary, processed carbohydrates at night.
- Customize starchy carbohydrates for your specific needs (see next chapter).
- Nonstarchy vegetables are OK anytime (as long as they are not smothered in cream sauce!).

Read on to see how modifying carbohydrate intake and glycemic index helped one of my patients finally lose the extra pounds she had been carrying for years, despite adhering to a vigorous exercise routine.

* * *

DVJ is a beautiful African-American woman—inspiring, and incredibly successful—who came to see me three months before her fiftieth birthday. She was exercising five to seven days a week and eating a generally healthy diet but had struggled for years to lose the extra thirty pounds or so that she was carrying. In the past she had had modest success with Weight Watchers, Diet Center, NutriSystem, and Atkins but always seemed to regain the weight she worked so hard to lose. Her cholesterol and blood sugar were normal, but her good cholesterol was low, and she had both high blood pressure and a waist size greater than thirty-five inches. She fit the criteria for metabolic syndrome, so I suggested that she cut back significantly on her starchy carbohydrate intake. Using the Carbohydrate Calculator that I developed, I recommended she aim for three to four servings of starch per day and increase her protein slightly to make sure she did not get hungry.

In her first week, she lost five pounds, half of which was water. She told me that though the first few days of cutting back on starchy carbohydrates had been difficult, it quickly became easier, and she was not getting hungry. She had even cut back slightly on her workouts due to a demanding work schedule. Over the next month, she did not lose very much weight, but her body fat was consistently dropping, so I assured her that things were moving in the right direction. I also encouraged her to pay more attention to the way her clothes were fitting than to the number on the scale. After two months, she lost ten pounds and was feeling great. She noticed that when she had bread or higher-sugar fruit, her blood sugar seemed "off," so she cut most of the bread and crackers from her diet and ate mainly beans and low-carb tortillas for her daily starches. She also felt better sticking to lower-sugar fruit, like apples and berries.

After another month she had lost five and a half more pounds, but her energy was not optimal. I urged her to increase her healthy carbohydrates on workout days, as she had cut back to one to two starches a day. Her energy improved, and she lost another five pounds over the next two months. At this point, her weight loss slowed considerably and hovered around the same level for about a month. I encouraged her to vary both the intensity and duration of her workouts and the carbohydrate level in her diet. The changes seemed to help, and she lost another six pounds over the next two months. Down by more than twenty-five pounds, she was now at the lowest weight that she had been in ten-plus years, but she still believed she would feel better ten pounds lighter.

The next week, stress at work led to a few overeating episodes, and her weight increased approximately one pound. She refused to be discouraged and simply got right back on track and came in the next week, down several pounds.

The following week, she left for a ten-day cruise, and I must admit that I was a bit concerned. Cruises are, without a doubt, among the most challenging of eating situations. Much to my surprise, she came back a month later, minus another three and a half pounds. She had walked a lot during the cruise and had endeavored to make good food choices and trade-offs, opting for dessert only if she was going dancing and minimizing bread intake. At this point, down thirty-three pounds (and slightly below her initial goal weight), she hit a plateau, and, despite all our best efforts, her weight refused to budge, so we began to focus on maintenance instead.

Since then, she has managed to drop a couple more pounds, but those few pounds inevitably return. However, she never allows herself to gain more than two or three pounds without taking immediate action. We continue to periodically experiment with different diet and exercise strategies to try to get rid of those last few pounds, but it is much more challenging for women during and after menopause. Besides, she looks incredible. I am thrilled that she continues to maintain her thirty-plus-pound weight loss despite a busy social life, frequent travel, and a demanding job.

THE BUSY PERSON'S PRINCIPLE 4:
PORTION SIZE *DOES* MATTER MOST OF THE TIME

Any "expert" who insists that portion size does not matter at all for weight loss is most likely not really an expert. I am not suggesting that portion size is the only relevant factor, but we can't minimize or ignore the direct association between America's expanding waistline and the increase in the size of everything, including plates, sodas, burgers, bagels, and buckets of popcorn. Research has shown that if a person is served a larger portion, he or she will eat more without being aware of eating more, without feeling more full, and without eating less at the next meal.[14, 15] Clearly, portion size matters. But with the supersizing of everything in America, what can the average person do that requires relatively little time and effort to control portions? Here are a few suggestions.

Relearning Portion Sizes

First, you should spend a little time retraining your eye to correct portion sizes. Get a set of measuring cups, spoons, and an inexpensive food scale, and experiment with the foods you eat most often. Put a measuring cup in your cereal box or nut jar. Throw that piece of cheese that you mindlessly snack on before dinner onto the scale for a reality check. Measure the amount of oil you use in salad dressing or cooking. You will probably be surprised at how much you are eating. It is incredible how much small changes add up. An extra half cup of cereal, two tablespoons of nuts, and a second tablespoon of oil add up to almost 300 calories. If you did that on a daily basis, you could gain almost thirty-six pounds a year. Familiarize yourself with portion sizes of starches and fats because these are the foods that people tend to overindulge in the most. I can safely say that in all my years of practicing, I have never had a patient not lose weight due to eating too many green vegetables.

To make things even simpler and less time-consuming, try to stick with foods that are naturally portion controlled. Have an English muffin instead of a huge bagel or muffin. Buy one-ounce bags of nuts, or put a quarter cup into a zip-lock bag, so when you reach into your desk or purse, you grab only one serving. Choose string cheese instead of slicing cheese from a block. Try eating on smaller plates to reduce your portion sizes and drinking out of taller or thinner glasses so your portions appear larger. And when dining out, automatically take half of your meal home (this saves time making lunch or dinner the next day), or share a meal with a friend. You may even order an appetizer for an entrée, as appetizer portions are usually more appropriate. (But stay away from the fried or fatty choices, like cheese sticks and potato skins.)

If you have a hard time controlling portions or you are the type of person who needs a larger volume of food to be satisfied, it is important to understand the concept of *energy density* of food. Lowering the energy density of your diet will allow you to eat fewer calories without having to watch portions as closely. This concept is the basis of several popular weight-loss books and has been championed by researcher Dr. Barbara Rolls, who has done extensive research into the energy density of food and its role in total caloric intake. A food's energy density represents the number of calories per gram (weight measurement).

Protein and carbohydrates have four calories per gram, and fat has nine calories per gram. Therefore, higher-fat foods such as nuts, cheese, oils, butter, salad dressing, cream, and sauces have a high energy density. Foods with high water content—fruits, vegetables, low-fat dairy, and soups—have a low energy density since water has no calories per gram. Conversely, dry foods like pretzels, chips, and cookies have a high energy density even if they are low-fat because they contain no water. Finally, since fiber is essentially calorie free, higher-fiber foods like fruits, vegetables, and whole grains also tend to have a low energy density.

It is also important to consider the *physical density* of food.

For example, compare the physical density of a bagel to an English muffin or slice of bread. The bagel is much denser, has twice the calories of an English muffin, and has four times the calories of a slice of bread. Similarly, compare the density of a brownie to a piece of cake. A very small brownie has the same number of calories as a larger piece of cake.

Energy Density, Portions, and Calories

Does energy density really matter? In a recent study, researchers showed that the combined effect of eating higher energy-density foods plus larger portions led people to eat 56 percent more food per meal without compensating at their next meal.[16] With results like this, it is not hard to see how our country's jumbo-size portions of tasty, energy-dense foods have played a role in our nation's obesity epidemic. However, energy density is not the whole story. After all, most Americans realize the importance of eating more fruits and vegetables, yet few are successful at weight loss. In my opinion, lowering the energy density of the diet represents only part of the weight-loss solution. The complete solution involves combining the benefits of a lower energy-density diet (less need for portion control, more filling) with the advantages of a diet centered around protein-based meals and snacks (less hunger, metabolic edge, stable blood sugar) to achieve permanent weight-loss success.

Lowering the Energy Density of Your Diet

Here are a few ways to decrease the energy density of your diet. For more ideas, take a look at Dr. Barbara Rolls's latest book, *The Volumetrics Eating Plan*.[17]

- Put vegetables in everything: eggs, soups, sandwiches, pasta dishes, rice dishes, etc.
- Start meals with broth-based soups, or salads without high-fat toppings and dressings.
- Make dressings and sauces out of nonfat yogurt instead of oil.
- Limit quantities of dry, salty snacks (chips, pretzels, nuts) if you have portion-control issues.
- Limit yourself to one medium- or high-density item per snack and a maximum of two per meal (for example, don't eat cheese and nuts for a snack—have just one of them, and eat it with a piece of fruit instead).

THE BUSY PERSON'S PRINCIPLE 5:
BUILD ACTIVITY INTO YOUR LIFE PERMANENTLY

I will go into much more detail about exercise in Chapter Four, but it is critical to understand that exercise not only plays a part in successful weight loss by helping to maintain your muscle mass and metabolism, but it is even more important for successful weight maintenance and optimal health. Even if you don't achieve your goal weight, research shows that it is healthier to be fit and overweight than to be normal weight and inactive.[18] Exercise helps lower blood pressure, blood sugar, and cholesterol, even if you don't lose a lot of weight. It can also help manage stress and depression. (Remember the term *runner's high*? Ever experienced it?)

The key is to develop an exercise strategy that is time efficient and that you will stick with for the long-term. Don't worry about the heart-rate charts, government guidelines, or your personal trainer's insistence that you get to the gym five times a week for an hour to achieve the results you desire. Your approach must fit into your life, not be forced in. My goal in Chapter Four is to help you find a way to get moving regularly and permanently.

> Don't worry about the heart-rate charts, government guidelines, or your personal trainer's insistence that you get to the gym five times a week for an hour to achieve the results you desire. Your approach must fit into your life, not be forced in.

THE BUSY PERSON'S PRINCIPLE 6:
DITCH THE ALL-OR-NOTHING MENTALITY

This may seem obvious, but I have seen numerous people fail at weight loss or fall short of their goals because of this deeply ingrained mentality. Remember that the suggestions I present throughout this book are *recommendations*, not rules set in stone. Some of them will work well for you; some won't. There will be days when you are able to follow them closely. There will be others when you are so busy or tired or stressed that you don't have the energy to do anything right (though most of my patients, when prodded, admit to doing *something* right on these days!). That's OK. Give yourself permission to make a few less-than-perfect choices occasionally, and for goodness' sake, don't beat yourself up about it. Just try to make the best choices you can, the majority of the time, and get back on track as soon as possible if you slip up for a meal, a day, or even a week.

Don't skip your workout because you only have twenty minutes instead of the hour that you had planned. If you don't have time to exercise or get to the gym habitually, do what you can to move your body and get your heart rate up at home, any chance that you get. Don't blow an entire meal simply because you didn't have time for an afternoon snack, got to the restaurant famished, and ate a slice or two of bread. Just try to make even better choices the rest of the meal or the next day. If you expect yourself to be perfect, you will fail, guaranteed. No one is perfect all the time. I skip my workouts when I get overcommitted. I *love* chocolate-chip cookies and pizza, and I indulge on occasion. The key is to do the best you can and to be consistent.

My favorite quote (attributed to Mary Pickford) that I often share with patients who have had a bad day or week is "Failure lies not in falling down but in *staying* down." Think about that, and consider repeating it to yourself when you feel you have "fallen down" in your weight-loss program by overindulging. As long as you try to be consistent and are making more good choices than bad, you will succeed in the long run!

THE BUSY PERSON'S PRINCIPLE 7:
ALWAYS HAVE A PLAN

You wouldn't go on a vacation without one. You wouldn't start a new business without one. You probably don't even go out for a night on the town without one. But it is amazing how many people who are trying to lose weight constantly find themselves in eating situations without one—a plan, that is. This may sound like basic common sense, but I can't tell you how many of my patients get off track because they don't plan ahead. This does not mean that you have to figure out exactly what you are going to eat for every meal and snack every day of the week. Some people do better with that type of planning, but most busy people don't do well with such a rigid approach. What I mean by having a plan is to think through eating (and exercise) options ahead of time. This means not only planning for healthy eating, but also planning for indulgences too. If you plan for them correctly, they won't derail your diet.

For example, if your job keeps you on the road most of the time, have a piece of fruit, some nuts, or a protein bar handy in the car at all times. And get to know the healthy fast-food or fast-casual restaurant options on your regular route or near your office. If you know you are going to a big dinner party or work dinner, try to eat fewer starchy carbohydrates and fats during the day to give yourself a little flexibility at dinner. If you are going to a holiday bash, decide in advance if you are going to have a little dessert or maybe an extra glass of wine instead. Or maybe your friend makes the best bread this side of the Mississippi, and you know you can't resist a slice or two. Plan that into your day by skipping the sandwich at lunch and having a salad with chicken instead. If you are going to a conference, assume that the food options may not be the most favorable. Try to start with a healthy breakfast, and have a wholesome snack on hand when the afternoon "cookie break" comes around.

It is also critical to plan to shop at least one day a week to make sure you have lots of healthy food options available at home and at the office, if necessary. The key is to not just let your meals "happen" but to have some type of plan for almost any eating situation in which you may find yourself. This can be done with very little effort utilizing the meal ideas, dining-out guide, and shopping lists provided later on in this book. The small amount of time you spend planning will translate into big results in weight loss and maintenance.

Now that you understand the basics about the Busy Person's Diet, it's time to learn how to put it into practice and design a program specifically suited to you. The next chapter will get you started at customizing your weight-loss program and will go into more detail about food categories and choices. I know this may seem like a lot of information, especially for someone with no time to lose, but trust me, taking the time to learn the basics and build the ideal weight-loss program for you will pay off in the end and really increase your chances of permanent weight loss!

The Busy Person's Basic Principles Summary

Principle 1:
Try to eat some form of protein with every meal and snack
   It maximizes metabolism.
   It stabilizes blood sugar.
   It controls hunger.

Principle 2:
Try to eat every three to four hours
   It controls hunger.
   It stabilizes blood sugar.

Principle 3:
Eat the right carbohydrates in the right quantity at the right time
   Eat mainly low-glycemic-load carbohydrates.
   Minimize starches at night.
   Customize carbohydrates for your unique situation.

Principle 4:
Portion size *does* matter most of the time
   Build portion control into your life.
   Lower the energy density of your diet.

Principle 5:
Build activity into your life permanently
   Make exercise excuse-proof and time-efficient.
   Increase lifestyle activity.

Principle 6:
Ditch the all-or-nothing mentality
Maintain a big-picture, lifestyle-based approach.

Principle 7:
Always have a plan
Never face eating occasions completely unprepared.
Plan indulgences.
Plan exercise or activity.

TWO

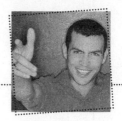

The Busy Person's Guide Customized for You

In working with people all day, every day, who are trying to lose weight, one of the most important things I have learned is that there is no one-size-fits-all for weight loss. It's true that genetics plays a significant role in your ability to lose weight. But so do many other important factors, including where you carry your weight (hips/thighs vs. waist); medical issues, like abnormal blood sugar and high cholesterol; food preferences; lifestyle (travel, entertaining, young kids); job type (seated, standing, labor); daily general activity level; and exercise preferences/abilities. To be successful in the long-term, a weight-loss plan must take into account as many of these variables as possible. This is not easy to do without seeing you in my office, but I have devised an approach very

37

similar to my daily approach with patients, to help you customize your weight-loss program.

DETERMINE YOUR READINESS TO LOSE WEIGHT

Before we begin customizing your weight-loss program, try to determine your weight-loss readiness and take a good look at your current life circumstances (no, just buying this book does not indicate readiness though it's a good start). Many people fail at weight loss not because they have chosen the wrong diet but because they are just not ready to do what it takes both mentally and physically. They set themselves up for failure before they even start. There will never be a perfect time to start a diet, but even for busy people there are better times than others. See how one of my most successful patients initially failed at weight loss because she just was not ready.

● ● ●

HN is not only one of my most successful patients but also a great example of the importance of readiness and motivation to lose weight. She initially came to see me one October with the goal of losing thirty pounds by her wedding, the next summer. She was finishing school and lived a chaotic, disorganized life. Her eating and exercise were erratic at best, and she did not seem interested in trying to figure out how to improve her eating habits. She blamed her fast-food diet and sporadic workouts on her busy and stressful schedule. She continued seeing me for about two months, during which time she went up and down the same three or four pounds several times. She would binge eat, and then binge exercise. She was not recording what she ate and was going for hours without eating. After Christmas I did not hear from her, so I decided not to contact her.

A year and a half later, HN called and asked if she could come back to see me. She had finished school and gotten married as planned the previous July. She had also gone on to gain fifty pounds more than when she originally came to me. I could hear the desperation in her voice, and since her life seemed to have settled down a bit, we made an appointment for the following week. This time, she really listened to what I was saying and began planning her eating and exercise ahead of time and writing in a journal regularly. Her husband, a chef, was also supportive and tried to prepare healthier options when he was home. Still, she found it was often easier to do her own thing when it came to meals.

She slowly began to exercise regularly, which is not easy for someone who is eighty pounds overweight. She often found herself winded walking routes that used to be effortless. After six weeks she lost an amazing twenty-one pounds and began feeling less dependent on the number on the scale each week. She still lacked confidence in her eating, and if she made one or two less-than-perfect choices during the week, she came in expecting the scale to be up. It wasn't. She had eaten well 80 to 90 percent of the time. After another six weeks and an additional sixteen-pound weight loss, she realized that she did not have to be perfect to lose weight. She also decided to exercise more and began playing tennis and hiking with her husband on weekends.

During the next five months, she continued to expand her exercise regimen to include longer cardio sessions, weights, and even spinning classes at the gym she had joined. But she got nervous when she started to feel hungrier. I assured her that this was a normal consequence of exercising more and that she should adjust her food intake upward slightly. I also told her to eat a piece of fruit before more vigorous workouts.

After eight months, HN lost a total of sixty pounds and dropped her body fat more than 10 percent. She has a totally new attitude toward eating and exercise and is confident in her ability to keep it off for good!

Defining Your Motivation

First, it is important to define your motivation for losing weight. Why do you really want to lose? For your upcoming class reunion? To please a spouse or parent? To meet a potential mate or become a parent? To fit into the jeans you wore in high school? To feel good about yourself? To be a role model for your children? For health concerns, current or future? Take some time to identify your motive for losing weight. Write down a few reasons. People with short-term or external reasons for losing weight, like a reunion or to please a spouse, are often not successful in the long-term because they fail to adopt the lifestyle changes critical for long-term weight loss. If your reasons are external or short-range, perhaps you may benefit from thinking more internally.

Health reasons are often the strongest motivation for weight loss, but most people, including many doctors, do not truly appreciate the strength of the association between obesity and disease or do not believe in the ability of weight loss to treat or decrease the risk of many obesity-related diseases. While there is undoubtedly a genetic component to many of the diseases listed in the following table, poor eating habits, inactivity, and obesity play a huge role as well. If you think your weight is not affecting your health, take a look at all the medical complications of obesity listed here. If you have a family history of any of these conditions or currently suffer from one or more of these, you will benefit from weight loss. Even a 5- to 10-percent weight loss can significantly lower your risk for many of these diseases.

MEDICAL COMPLICATIONS OF OBESITY

Heart disease	Infertility
High cholesterol	Polycystic ovarian syndrome
Diabetes	Arthritis
Metabolic syndrome	Cancer
Stroke	Depression
Sleep apnea	Kidney stones
Fatty liver disease	Alzheimer's
Gout	

If you are trying to lose weight to please someone else, be honest with yourself. Is this really important to *you*? Would you feel better about yourself if you lost weight? Would you be more confident? Try to find a reason to do this *for yourself*, and you will experience more lasting success. Take some time here to list your reasons for wanting to lose weight and the negative consequences of being overweight that apply to you. It is a good idea to refer back to these periodically during both weight loss and maintenance.

Reasons I Want to Lose Weight:

1._____

2._____

3._____

Negative Consequences of My Being Overweight:

1._____

2._____

3._____

If you don't believe that weight loss can considerably impact your health, read on to learn how one of my patients experienced an incredible drop in cholesterol with weight loss alone, despite her doctor's desire to put her on medication.

● ● ●

SP is an attorney in her mid-fifties. Less than five feet tall, she was carrying an extra forty pounds on her petite frame and had very high cholesterol. Despite the extra weight, she was very active and took spinning classes at the gym regularly, but her busy schedule made eating a challenge. She ate most lunches and dinners out or had takeout at her desk. She told me her weight had always fluctuated but had increased even more after menopause. Since carbohydrates were her favorite food, she had not tried to reduce them in the past to lose weight. Her typical eating day consisted of a bagel and latte for breakfast, a restaurant salad and main course for lunch, and a frozen dinner or takeout at night, often followed by a midnight snack of milk and cookies.

Because of her demanding schedule, SP would only be able to see me monthly instead of every week or two, as most of my patients do. Most patients with infrequent visits are not as successful, but I agreed to meet with her once a month and see how things progressed. I started out by making sure that she had lean protein beginning with breakfast and appreciably reducing her starchy carbohydrates. After a month, she came back in, and—despite reporting that she had a hard time counting food group servings—to my surprise she had lost four and a half pounds.

She, too, was surprised at how easily the weight was coming off and that she was not having cravings for carbs as she feared. She began bringing her snacks and an easy lunch— a premade salad from a speciality grocer like Trader Joe's— to work instead of eating takeout at her desk.

After three months, she was down 14 ½ pounds. Prior to getting on the scale each month, she told me she was sure she had not lost weight, because she did not feel as if she was on a diet. "That is my goal," I explained on a regular basis, with a chuckle. It always amazes me that people think they have to suffer and feel as though they are "on a diet" when attempting to lose weight. After about six months, down 21 pounds, she began coming in every two months, and though the weight loss slowed considerably, it never stopped, much to her wonder and mine.

After slightly more than a year, and down 35 ½ pounds, SP finally had her cholesterol rechecked, and the results were astounding. Her total cholesterol dropped 22 percent, triglycerides were down 41 percent, bad cholesterol was down 31 percent, and her good cholesterol was exactly the same! Her eating habits had become completely "second nature," and she actually continued losing relatively effortlessly beyond her initial goal weight.

Timing Is Everything—Evaluating the Next Two Months of Your Life

Another important factor in determining your readiness is to evaluate the next couple months of your life. This time period is critical in any weight-loss program as it takes a month or two for new habits to form and for the program to become "second nature." Are you moving? Starting a new job? Taking an extended trip that you have been planning for two years? Entering the holiday season with a packed social schedule? If you are making any major changes or have significant obligations in the next few months, it may not be the best time to put tremendous effort into losing weight. While you may have the time, you may not have the mental capacity or be in the right environment to lose weight. It will take a little thought, planning, and organization (not necessarily time) to figure out a system that works for you.

While the Busy Person's Diet can be done anywhere, with minimal time and resources, some situations (like travel to foreign countries, houses turned upside down, moves to new cities, stressful new jobs, and nightly holiday parties) can make things more difficult and add more stress to your life than it's worth at this point. You may be better off waiting until things normalize a bit. Or you could read the book now with the intent of picking up a few tips and working slowly toward adopting a healthier lifestyle and perhaps simply maintaining rather than losing weight, until your life settles down. Timing and motivation are important components of successful, long-term weight loss.

DEFINING YOUR GOAL WEIGHT AND RATE OF WEIGHT LOSS

Once you have evaluated your timing and motivation, the next step toward a personalized and permanent weight-loss plan is to define (1) a realistic goal weight and (2) a sensible rate of weight loss. I know you want to get back to your college weight *yesterday*, but if you don't put a little thought into these two questions, you may be setting yourself up to fail. Understanding your reality is an important part of successful weight loss. I see so many people who begin a weight-loss program with completely unrealistic expectations. This quickly leads to disappointment and a sense of failure if they are not losing weight as quickly as they would like to or if they hit a plateau, pounds away from their goal.

Setting Realistic Expectations
for Your Rate of Weight Loss

Let's discuss the rate of weight loss first. One of the biggest issues I regularly face with my patients is convincing them of what is a realistic and appropriate weight-loss rate. Are you hoping that, if you work very hard, you will lose twenty pounds in the next month, before your trip to Mexico? If so, stop now. This is not a reality TV show, where you can exercise six hours a day and not focus on anything but weight loss. Under most circumstances, you simply cannot lose weight that quickly, and if you do, you are probably losing a significant amount of muscle, water, and even bone. Take a look at the math in the following box for a reality check on weight loss. After reviewing the information, you will understand why it is very difficult for women to lose more than one to two pounds of fat per week and for men to lose more than two to three pounds of fat per week.

CALCULATION FOR LOSS OF TWO TO FOUR POUNDS OF FAT PER WEEK

1 pound of fat = 3,500 calories

To lose 1 pound of fat per week = 1 x 3,500 = 3,500-calorie total weekly deficit

To lose 2 pounds of fat in one week = 2 x 3,500 = 7,000-calorie total weekly deficit

To lose 4 pounds of fat in one week = 4 x 3,500 = 14,000-calorie total weekly deficit

Assume the average 150-pound woman needs about 1,800–2,200 calories per day.

Assume the average 200-pound man needs about 2,200–2,600 calories per day.

Unrealistic Rate of Weight Loss

For a 150-pound woman to lose 4 pounds of fat per week, she would need a 14,000-calorie total weekly deficit.

14,000 / 7 = 2,000-calorie deficit per day
Eat nothing daily with no exercise

Eat 1,000 calories per day and burn 1,000 calories

Eat 2,000 calories per day and burn 2,000 calories

For a 200-pound man to lose 4 pounds of fat in one week, he would need a 14,000-calorie total weekly deficit.

14,000 / 7 = 2,000 calorie deficit per day

Eat 500 calories per day without exercise

Eat 1,500 calories per day and burn 1,000 calories

Eat 2,500 calories per day and burn 2,500 calories

Realistic Rate of Weight Loss

For a 150-pound woman to lose 2 pounds of fat per week, she would need a 7,000-calorie total weekly deficit.

7,000 / 7 = 1,000 calorie deficit per day

Eat 1,000 calories per day without exercising

Eat 1,250 calories per day and burn 250 calories

Eat 1,500 calories per day and burn 500 calories

For a 200-pound man to lose 2 pounds of fat per week, he would need a 7,000-calorie total weekly deficit.

7,000 / 7 = 1,000 calorie deficit per day

Eat 1,500 calories per day without exercising

Eat 1,750 calories per day and burn 250 calories

Eat 2,000 calories per day and burn 500 calories

SETTING A REALISTIC GOAL WEIGHT

Now let's move on to your goal weight. Are you hoping to get down to the weight that you were in college, before the three kids, mortgage, and full-time job? If so, you may want to reevaluate. What did it take to get and stay there back then? Do you really have the time or energy at this point in your life? Is it worth the sacrifices? For some people, particularly younger men, weight loss may not be that challenging, and you may easily lose several pounds a week and get down to your high-school-wrestling weight. For most others, the realities of life, such as travel, children, demanding jobs, sick parents or spouses, and even genetics, require more realistic goals.

Speaking of genetics, let me briefly explain the role it plays in weight loss. Research suggests that genetics plays a major role in obesity (anywhere from 30 to 70 percent),[1] but this does not mean that you are destined to be overweight if one (or both) of your parents has a weight problem. It does mean that you are probably more susceptible to environmental factors, such as increased food availability, larger portions, and better-tasting cuisine, which lead to weight gain. You may feel hungrier more frequently than someone who does not struggle with weight. Or perhaps you don't feel full as easily, so you eat slightly more when you are served the same amount of food as a thinner person. Or your body may not handle carbohydrates as efficiently as it could, causing you to more easily store excess carbs as fat. The bottom line is, whatever role genetics plays, you still have some control. You may have to eat a little less or a little differently and exercise a little bit more, but permanent weight loss is possible for the great majority of overweight people. I am not saying that you can have the figure of a supermodel or pro athlete if you work hard enough, but you can have a strong, fit, healthy body—if you are committed.

It is also important to remember that metabolism does slow as we age. A significant cause of this drop in metabolism is a decrease in muscle mass, some of which is preventable through strength training. Some muscle loss, though, is simply the consequence of aging and physiological changes in the body, both of which are beyond your control. So factor age into your goal setting too!

Now that you understand what is realistic, try to choose a weight (or clothing size) that you feel you can comfortably maintain. You will probably never weigh what you weighed in high school again, or what you weighed before you had children and could devote hours a day to exercise. Try to remember a time, weight, or size in your life when you felt comfortable and that was not a huge daily struggle to maintain. I often encourage my patients to focus more on clothing size than weight, since favorable changes in body composition (increased muscle-to-fat ratio) can increase your weight slightly, but decrease your pant size. And gaining muscle should never be seen as a bad thing, since it helps with long-term weight loss by increasing or maintaining metabolism.

If you have more than thirty pounds to lose, consider setting several smaller weight-loss goals. Start with a goal of 5 to 10 percent of your body weight. This amount of weight loss alone can have a very large impact on your overall health. Once you have attained that goal, reassess the situation.

How do you feel? How is your health? How hard was it for you to reach this goal? Are you still motivated to lose more, or do you feel more comfortable maintaining at this weight for a period of time? Whatever you do, don't stop focusing on your eating and exercise. But try to be realistic with yourself.

Take some time here to figure and write down a few goals:

Starting Weight: _____

5 Percent Weight Loss =
    Starting Weight x .05 = _____

10 Percent Weight Loss =
    Starting Weight x .10 = _____

Weight I Would Be Content With = _____

My Ultimate-Goal Weight = _____

You may want to share these goals with a close friend, family member, or even your physician. Making your goals public may help you stay on track or give you added motivation to succeed.

Now that you have defined a realistic goal weight and a few mini target weights along the way, take a little time to write down three things that you are most looking forward to when you reach any one of these weights. Try to put some thought into these three things, and really imagine yourself at these weights. You may want to refer back to these when you find motivation dropping or hit a rough spot in your weight-loss efforts.

What I am looking forward to most when I reach my goal weight:

1._____

2._____

3._____

One final note: You do not have to define a goal weight. It is completely acceptable to begin your weight-loss program with the goal of losing an undefined amount of weight, fitting into a specific pair of pants, or just becoming healthier and more active. If you are the type of person who has been obsessed your entire life with the scale, this may allow you to focus more on positive changes than the number on the scale. Similarly, if you are someone who is not really focused on weight but rather on health, defining health-related goals may work just as well or even better.

The Importance of Customizing Carbohydrates

Americans are confused about carbohydrates. With the passing of the low-carb diet craze, most Americans realize that dramatically cutting carbohydrates is neither healthy nor realistic over the long-term. You may last a few months without a piece of bread or a cookie, but good luck getting through the holidays, vacations, or a dinner party at your mother-in-law's. While dramatically cutting carbs is not the solution, limiting carbohydrates is important, especially in the nearly 70 percent of overweight Americans who have a condition called *metabolic syndrome*.[2]

> You may last a few months without a piece of bread or a cookie, but good luck getting through the holidays, vacations, or a dinner party at your mother-in-law's.

Metabolic syndrome is not a disease but rather a group of symptoms including high blood pressure, low good cholesterol, high triglycerides, high blood sugar, and the tendency to carry extra weight mainly around the waist rather than evenly distributed on the entire body (being apple-shaped instead of pear-shaped). If you have three or more of these symptoms, you probably have metabolic syndrome, and both heart disease and diabetes are strongly associated with metabolic syndrome. But if you think you may have metabolic syndrome, there is no need to panic and run to the emergency room. The best treatment is diet and exercise. Research indicates that people with metabolic syndrome lose weight more effectively when they reduce carbohydrates, especially highly processed, sugary, or starchy carbohydrates.[3]

In addition to the absence or presence of metabolic syndrome, your weight, age, and activity level influence how many carbohydrates you need for optimal weight loss. To help you figure out the level of carbohydrates that is best for you, I have developed a Carbohydrate Calculator worksheet. The worksheet will help you determine the amount of starchy carbohydrates that you can consume and still lose weight. While the calculator works for most, I have seen enough patients to know that it does not work for everyone. If you are not losing weight after one or two weeks on the program, and you carry your weight mainly around your midsection, or you are peri- or postmenopausal, try cutting your starch by one until you begin to lose. If you find that you absolutely cannot live on the number of starches calculated, add one or two in place of another food type or exercise more to "earn" an additional starch.

As you lose weight, the amount of starch you can consume may change. Some people, particularly men who carry their weight around the middle, can actually slightly *increase* their starchy carbohydrates, especially if they also increase their exercise levels significantly and gain muscle. Others, especially smaller or peri- and postmenopausal women, may need to cut their starchy carbohydrates slightly as they lose weight, to continue reducing. You will have to experiment somewhat to figure out what works best for you, but you should redo the worksheet as you reach your interim weight-loss goals (5 percent, 10 percent, and so on) or if you hit a plateau that you are unable to break through after a few weeks.

The worksheet will be the most accurate if you see your doctor and figure out if you have high or high normal blood sugar, high triglycerides (blood fat), and low good cholesterol (HDL). If this is not possible, you can always measure your own waist, go to a pharmacy and take your own blood pressure, and figure out your family history of high cholesterol or diabetes (a strong family history suggests that you are at risk).

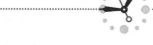

CARBOHYDRATE CALCULATOR WORKSHEET

Female Calculator

Start with 4 starches.

Add 1 starch if you are less than 20 years old, and subtract 1 if you are more than 50 years old. _____

Metabolic Syndrome

High blood pressure

High normal/high blood sugar

High triglycerides

Waist greater than 35 inches

Low good cholesterol

Subtract 1 starch if you have diabetes, have three out of five signs of metabolic syndrome, or consider your body type apple-shaped. _____

Evaluate activity level with the chart below:

Subtract 1 if you have low activity. _____
Do not change if you have moderate activity. _____
Add 1 if you have high activity. _____

Based on your weight:

Subtract 1 if you weigh <150 pounds. _____
Do not change if you weigh 150 to 200 pounds. _____
Add 1 if you weigh between 201 and 250 pounds. _____
Add 2 if you weigh >250 pounds. _____

The total represents the maximum number of servings of starchy carbohydrates you should eat on a daily basis to lose weight. If your answers to any of the questions change (for example, you lose weight, your waist size decreases, or you exercise more), recalculate your total daily starch exchanges.

Male Calculator

Start with 6 starches.
Add 1 starch if you are less than 20 years old, and subtract 1 if you are more than 40 years old. _____

> ### *Metabolic Syndrome*
> High blood pressure
> High normal/high blood sugar
> High triglycerides
> Waist greater than 35 inches
> Low good cholesterol

Subtract 1 starch if you have diabetes, have three out of five signs of metabolic syndrome, or consider your body type apple-shaped. _____

Evaluate activity level with the chart below:

Subtract 1 if you have low activity. _____
Do not change if you have moderate activity. _____
Add 1 if you have high activity. _____

Based on your weight:

Do not change if you weigh <250 pounds. _____
Add 1 if you weigh between 251 and 300 pounds. _____
Add 2 if you weigh >300 pounds. _____

The total represents the maximum number of servings of starchy carbohydrates you should eat on a daily basis to lose weight. If your answers to any of the questions change (for example, you lose weight, your waist size decreases, or you exercise more), recalculate your total daily starch exchanges.

Activity Level	Description
Low	Low-activity job (such as desk job) and/or very light exercise program (such as 30 minutes light walking) 3 times per week or less
Moderate	Moderate-activity job (some standing required) and/or moderate exercise performed 4 to 5 times per week (30 minutes jogging/biking or 45–60 minutes fast walking)
High	High-activity job (construction worker) and/or moderately vigorous exercise more than 5 times per week (45–60 minutes of moderate-to-high intensity; can include walking hills, jogging, aerobics, spinning, swimming)

See how modifying carbohydrates helped one of my favorite long-term patients—and his wife—achieve a combined 130-pound weight loss!

● ● ●

VS is a local law enforcement officer. At five feet, seven inches, he was almost one hundred pounds overweight. In addition to struggling with routine physical activity on the job, he had high blood pressure, high cholesterol, and a strong family history of heart disease and diabetes. He first came to see me at the age of forty-eight and reported that he had been steadily gaining weight since his late twenties. He was finally ready to "regain control" of his diet and eating, he wrote when answering his weight and diet history question-naire. Despite his erratic schedule and long hours, he was walking four days a week, for at least an hour, with his wife, who also struggled with her weight. She had been very suc-cessful with Weight Watchers in the past but always seemed to regain the weight.

VS's eating wasn't really that bad when he came to see me. A typical day included a SlimFast bar at 5:30 AM; a sand-wich/apple/salad/cracker/cookies for lunch, between 1 and 3 PM; and a dinner of meat/vegetable/starch/salad between 7 and 8 PM, followed by ice cream, cookies, or candy at 9 PM. I decided to be a bit more aggressive at reducing VS's starchy carbohydrates initially since he had a large amount of weight to lose and met the criteria for metabolic syn-drome. He would lose weight more quickly, which would be motivating, but I strongly encouraged him to begin a weight-training program to maintain or improve his muscle mass. He got off to a great start, losing a remark-able fourteen pounds during his two weeks, most of which was fat. I told him not to expect such large weekly weight losses in the future, and I suggested that he add beans to dinner to slow down his weight loss a bit and make sure he did not risk losing muscle mass.

Over the holidays, he avoided tempting sweets and high-glycemic starches since he was doing so well on his weight-loss program. He came back in mid-January, down another 12 ½ pounds, which is the most weight any of my patients has ever lost over the holidays. At this point, his weight loss began to slow to a more reasonable rate, about two pounds a week. To keep himself motivated, he started wearing a pedometer to count his steps, and he challenged himself to break 10,000 steps as often as possible. After six months, he was down an impressive sixty pounds. At this point his wife hesitantly made an appointment to see me.

She was thrilled with her husband's weight loss and wanted to join in his success and lose the fifty pounds she had regained in the last ten years, but she was afraid that the program would not work as well for her. I explained to her that men lose weight more quickly than women due to greater muscle mass and a possible female hormone effect that causes many women to store fat more easily and lose it more slowly. MS was not a big eater, but she was a typical Weight Watchers veteran, who liked to "save" her calories for the evening instead of spreading calories evenly throughout the day. I see this practiced frequently in both male and female patients, and I call it "crescendo eating," resembling a music score that gets louder and louder as it progresses. I explained to MS that this was not the right way to fuel her body; she actually needed fewer calories at night, when she was the least active. I also detailed the importance of eating enough protein, something she had struggled with in the past, for both controlling hunger and maintaining muscle.

MS agreed to increase her protein intake, especially in the mornings, and watch her crescendo eating. After her first week, she lost three pounds and noticed an immediate increase in energy. She was amazed, because she was eating more than she had in the past. After five weeks she was down ten pounds, which wasn't much compared to her husband, but I assured her that she was doing terrific. She started adding resistance training to her exercise regimen, and her weight continued to slowly drop. At this point, I noticed that every time MS came in, she immediately told me everything that she felt she had done wrong that week. Since she was steadily losing weight, I tried to direct our visits toward the things that she was doing correctly instead and encouraged her to write in her food journal several things that she had done well each week.

After seeing me for about four months and losing twenty-two pounds, life got stressful for MS, but for the first time in her life, she wasn't reaching for sweets when she felt stressed. I could tell how empowered she felt by the control she had over her eating and was thrilled at her mental and physical progress. Meanwhile, her husband, VS, was now down sixty-seven pounds and was becoming a little less vigilant with his eating. They had only healthy foods in the house, but his portions were creeping up little by little, and he gained a little weight for the first time in seven months. After reviewing his food journal, I told him he needed to clean up his eating a bit and keep a closer eye on his portions, especially of higher-fat and dry snack foods, like nuts and soy chips. He agreed to watch the snacking and lost three and a half pounds by the next week.

Over the next few months, he lost another fifteen pounds, for a total weight loss of eighty-seven pounds. He was down to the smallest dose of blood pressure and cholesterol medication and had to be fitted for a new gun belt when he ran out of holes and it simply would not stay up anymore. At this point, his weight loss stopped, thirteen pounds short of his goal weight. For several months, including over the holidays, his weight did not budge. A back injury in early January was affecting his workouts, and his body did not seem to be responding anymore, so I suggested he take a break and focus on maintaining. I saw him every month or so for the next six months, and his weight was holding steady, so we decided to see each other three months later.

He returned three months later with an eight-pound weight gain. I asked what he thought was the problem, and he said he was eating more, especially salty snacks at night, and exercising less. He agreed to start using his journal again to record what he ate and to see me every few weeks until he was back on track. He is now back down near his lowest point and holding steady. His wife, MS, lost an additional twenty-seven pounds in the year since I stopped seeing her regularly, for a grand total of forty-nine pounds, one pound short of her goal weight, which she had last weighed fourteen years ago. Needless to say, with a total combined 132 pounds' weight loss, the two of them look and, more importantly, feel incredible. While they both had very different eating issues and took somewhat different approaches to my recommendations, they remain incredibly supportive of each other, and I'm confident that they have made the permanent lifestyle changes necessary to maintain their incredible weight loss for good.

LEARNING THE BASIC FOOD GROUPS

There are many different approaches to thinking about and categorizing food for the purpose of weight loss. Some programs require you to count points, blocks, calories, or grams of fat or carbohydrates. I prefer to focus more on the big picture when designing weight-loss programs and have found that giving my patients suggested daily ranges of each food group is the simplest approach. All foods are composed of at least one, if not several, of these food groups. I have tried to give as many examples in each category as possible, but this list is by no means exhaustive, and you will have to figure out a few things on your own by reading labels and doing some simple math.

I urge you to not overthink your eating or try to figure out exactly how to classify every bite that goes into your mouth. Focus more on the big picture, and you will be successful, without driving yourself crazy counting and calculating.

Starches _____. (Fill in the number you calculated using the Carbohydrate Calculator worksheet—this represents the average number of servings you should eat per day. You may choose to eat fewer initially to lose weight more quickly.)

Starches are the food group, along with fats (and perhaps alcohol for some), that should be monitored the most closely. Not only can these foods affect your blood sugar more than other foods, but they are generally much easier to overeat. As discussed earlier, it is important to choose the best quality starchy carbohydrates possible. The foods in this category can be a great source of heart-healthy soluble fiber, so pay attention to the fiber content when reading labels, and choose whole grains whenever possible. (To learn more about fiber, see the Focus on Fiber sidebar on pages 66–68.)

It is also important to consume most of your starchy carbohydrates earlier in the day and try not to eat them all at one meal. Finally, limit candy, sweets, and processed sugary snack foods as much as possible. Each item in the following list equals one starch serving. Your actual serving size may be larger or smaller. Calculate the number of starch servings according to your actual serving size.

ADOPTED FROM THE *OFFICIAL POCKET GUIDE TO DIABETIC EXCHANGES*

(American Diabetes Association, Inc.,
and the American Dietetic Association, 1997)

Overview

One starch serving = 1 slice bread or ½ cup of cereal, pasta, rice, or starchy vegetables (potatoes, corn, peas, beans)
  ▼ = less healthy starches
  ♥ = heart healthy starches

Serving Sizes

Bagel: ¼ deli or bagel shop variety, ½ frozen
♥ Barley/Bulgur: ¼ cup
▼ Biscuit: 1 small
Bread: 1 slice (opt for whole grain with a minimum of 2 grams fiber)
▼ Cake: 2-in. square unfrosted or 1-in. square frosted

♥ Cereal: ½ cup (serving size varies considerably. One serving = approximately 80 calories; aim for a minimum of 3 grams of fiber per serving and limit the sugar content)

▼ Chips: 1 oz. (12–18)

▼ Corn bread: 2-in. cube

▼ Cookie: 2 small

Couscous: ⅓ cup

English muffin: ½ (whole wheat best)

Flour: 3 tablespoons

Frozen yogurt/ice cream (fat-free, sugar-free): ½ cup

Granola (low-fat): ¼ cup

Graham crackers: 3

Grits: ½ cup

Matzoh: ¾ oz.

▼ Muffin: 1 ½ oz. (the average bakery or café muffin is 4 to 5 ounces and loaded with fat)

♥ Oatmeal: ½ cup cooked or ¼ cup raw (best if no sugar added)

Pancakes: (2) 4 in.

Pasta: ½ cup (whole wheat better)

Pita: (½) 6 in. (whole wheat best)

Popcorn (low-fat): 3 cups

Pretzels: ¾ oz.

Protein bar: 1 (starch servings in protein bars vary; just remember 15 grams of carbs = one starch)

Rice: ½ cup (brown rice is better)—for sushi lovers, 4 pieces = approximately ½ cup rice

Roll: 1 small dinner

Saltines: 6

Starchy vegetables:

♥ Beans/lentils: ½ cup (also count as 1 very lean protein, super high in fiber)

Corn: 1 medium corn cob or ½ cup cooked

Hummus: ⅓ cup

Peas (green, split, or black-eyed): ½ cup

Plantain: ½ cup

Potato: 1 small (3 oz.) or ½ cup cooked or mashed

Squash (acorn, butternut): 1 cup

Yam/sweet potato: ½ cup

▼ Stuffing: ⅓ cup

▼ Syrup: 1 tablespoon

Tortilla: (1) 6 in. (corn or flour)—low carbohydrate version = less than ½ starch per tortilla

Waffle: 4 ½ in.

Whole wheat crackers (low-fat): ¾ oz. (2–5)

Since starchy carbohydrates are an important source of fiber, now is a good time to briefly review the benefits of dietary fiber.

FOCUS ON FIBER

Why is fiber so important in your diet? Fiber is a type of carbo-hydrate obtained only from plant sources that humans cannot digest. Because it cannot be digested, it supplies essentially no calories. There are two types of dietary fiber: soluble and insoluble. Both are important for good health, weight loss, and disease prevention.

Insoluble fiber is found in whole grains, bran, whole wheat, beans, some fruits, and most vegetables. In the colon, insoluble fiber absorbs water, thereby softening stools, to help keep you regular. Low-carbohydrate diets often cause constipation, because they are low in insoluble fiber. A high-fiber diet may help lower your risk of colon cancer, especially a diet high in cereal fiber.

Soluble fiber, which is found in fruits (apples, strawberries, citrus), beans, seeds, cereals, oats, and barley, can help lower cholesterol by binding to the "bad" cholesterol in your bloodstream, preventing it from accumulating in your arteries. It can also help control blood sugar, as soluble fiber absorbs water in the stomach, forming a paste or gel that slows the absorption and digestion of food and leads to a more gradual rise in blood sugar. This can also make you feel full for a longer period of time, which can be helpful for weight loss.

Most high-fiber foods have a combination of soluble and insoluble fiber, so focus on increasing your overall fiber intake. Aim for 20 to 35 grams per day. If your diet is too low in fiber, increase your fiber intake slowly. If you increase too quickly, you will likely experience significant gas, constipation, and bloating. And make sure you drink plenty of water or you can become more constipated. It is important to choose mainly high-fiber starches to optimize your weight loss and health. Check out the following chart for some of the best (and worst) sources of fiber.

Cereal (1 cup, unless noted)	*Grams of Fiber*
Fiber One (½ cup)	14
Kellogg's All-Bran (½ cup)	10
Multi-Bran Chex, Kashi Good Friends (¾) cup	8
Raisin Bran	8
Spoon Size Shredded Wheat	6
Wheat Chex, Bran Flakes	5
Quaker Oats (cooked)	4
Cheerios or Wheaties	3
Kellogg's Corn Flakes	1
Special K or Rice Krispies	0

Grains and Pasta

Barley, whole wheat spaghetti	6
Brown rice	4
Buckwheat pancakes (4, 4 inch)	3
Couscous, macaroni, or spaghetti	2
White rice	1

Beans and Starchy Vegetables

Lentils (½ cup)	8
Pinto beans (½ cup)	7
Chickpeas, kidney beans (½ cup)	6
Green peas (1 cup)	4
Sweet potato	3
Corn (1 cup)	2

Let's continue with the rest of the basic food groups.

Dairy. One serving equals 1 cup or 8 oz. milk or yogurt. (Cottage cheese and cheese are listed in the protein category.) Aim for *two to three servings* per day.

Dairy has undergone a major image overhaul and has gained renewed popularity due to a few highly publicized studies that showed greater weight loss and fat loss in patients consuming high-dairy diets. The researchers speculate that the higher levels of calcium may help mobilize fat, and the lean protein in dairy may protect muscle.[4] While this research is not conclusive, low-fat (1 percent) or fat-free dairy is an important part of any healthy diet or weight-loss plan. There are, however, a few things to remember when choosing dairy.

It is essential to check the *sugar* content of yogurt. If high-fructose corn syrup or sugar is high on the list of ingredients, select a different brand. Always compare labels and choose lower-sugar options. Plain, fat-free, or low-fat yogurt is best, and you can add fresh or frozen fruit, Splenda, cinnamon, or vanilla extract. If you prefer flavored yogurts, vanilla yogurt is usually lower in sugar than fruit flavors. Fage's Total Greek Yogurt, Russian yogurt (Pavel), and Dannon Light 'n Fit are some of my favorite choices.

And though low-fat or nonfat milk are good sources of protein, calcium, and vitamin D, they are not calorie free. Those twice-a-day, jumbo, nonfat lattes may be slowing your weight loss considerably. If, like much of the world, you are lactose intolerant, consider taking Lactaid supplements with dairy or choosing lactose-free products. At the very least, take a daily calcium and vitamin D supplement.

Don't forget that dairy contains lean protein and can be considered a source of protein at meals or snacks.

Protein. *Men* should aim for *ten to fourteen ounces* of protein per day depending on their height and weight. *Women* should try to get *eight to twelve ounces* per day depending on their height and weight.

Recommendations are given in ounces, not servings. If you are taller or weigh more, stay on the higher end of the range. Smaller and less active people should stay on the lower end. It is not critical to consume exactly the recommended number of ounces per day. Just make sure to balance out your day; if you eat a large serving of protein at lunch, cut back at dinner. If you don't get much protein at breakfast, it is OK to have a bit more at your morning snack or at any other meal.

Remember that lean and very lean protein should be the foundation of most meals and snacks. Most of these foods are measured in ounces (cooked) with the exception of cottage cheese, eggs, and nuts. In general, aim for about *one to two ounces* of protein for *breakfast* and *snacks, three to five ounces* at *lunch*, and *three to six ounces* at *dinner*. Here are a few points to remember for optimal health and weight-loss success:

▪ Try to choose mainly those proteins that are low-fat and very low-fat. They contain up to 50 percent fewer calories per ounce than higher-fat proteins, so portion sizes are not as restricted.
▪ If you choose higher-fat proteins, you must decrease your portion size, and you may want to cut fat in other areas of your diet.

- In general, don't eat more than six to seven ounces of protein per meal. It is harder for your kidneys to get rid of larger amounts of protein.
- Always trim the fat or remove skin before or after cooking.
- Limit red meat and processed meats, like hot dogs and bologna, to twice a week or less, as they have been associated with a higher incidence of colon cancer.
- For approximating protein portions, a three-ounce serving is about the size of a deck of cards.
- Frequently include plant-based proteins for maximum health (beans, tofu, nuts).
- You may replace one dairy serving with two protein servings if you prefer to eat more protein, but try to include dairy proteins like cottage cheese or low-fat cheese in your diet.

Complete List of Proteins by Fat Quantity

Very low-fat:

1 oz. = 7 grams protein; less than 1 gram fat = 35 calories

Beans/Lentils: ½ cup (also count as 1 starch)

Buffalo

Clams

Cheese (fat free)

Chicken or Turkey (white meat, no skin)

Cornish hen (no skin)

Canned tuna in water

Cottage cheese (nonfat or low-fat): ¼ cup

Crab

Duck or Pheasant (no skin)
Egg substitute: ¼ cup
Egg whites (2)
Fish (cod, flounder, halibut, trout, tuna)
Hot dogs (fat free)
Lobster
Ostrich
Processed sandwich meat
    (low-fat or fat-free turkey, ham, etc.)
Scallops
Shrimp
Venison

Low-fat:
    1 oz. = 7 grams protein; 1–3 grams fat = 55 calories
    Beef: USDA Select or Choice, including round,
        sirloin, flank steak, tenderloin, roast (rib, chuck,
        rump), steak (T-bone, porterhouse, cubed), and
        ground round
    Cheese (low-fat)
    Chicken/Turkey (dark meat, no skin) or Chicken (white
        meat with skin)
    Herring (smoked not creamed)
    Goose
    Lamb: roast, chop, leg
    Oysters (6)
    Parmesan, grated: 2 tablespoons
    Pork: tenderloin, lean ham, or Canadian bacon
    Rabbit
    Salmon

Sardines (2)
Turkey, ground (extra lean)
Tuna (in oil, drained)
Tofu
Veal: lean chop, roast

Medium fat: 1 oz. = 7 grams protein; 3–5 grams fat = 75 calories (also count as ½ fat per ounce)

Beef: ground beef, meatloaf, veal, short ribs, prime
　　rib (trimmed), corned beef, meatballs, New
　　York strip
Cheese: feta, mozzarella, ricotta (¼ cup)
Chicken (dark meat with skin), fried chicken (with skin),
　　ground turkey
Egg (limit to one per day)
Fish, fried
Lamb: rib roast, ground
Low-fat or part-skim cheeses (ricotta, mozzarella, other
　　low-fat cheeses)
Pork: chops, top loin, or cutlets
Sausage (low-fat)
Tempeh: ¼ cup
Veal cutlet

High fat: 1 oz. = 7 grams protein; 5–8 grams fat = 100 calories (also count as 1 fat per ounce)

Ribs, brisket
Bacon: 3 slices
Cheese, regular: American, cheddar, Monterey Jack,
　　Swiss, brie

Hot dog, turkey or chicken (beef and pork are
    even worse)
*Nuts: ⅛ cup
*Peanut Butter: 1 tablespoon
Pepperoni (remember this the next time you
    order pizza!)
Pork: spareribs, ground pork, pork sausage
Sausage: bratwurst, Italian, Polish
Luncheon meats: bologna, pastrami, salami

*Note that peanut butter and nuts are made up of very healthy fats, are high in fiber, and are packed with nutrients, so long as you watch your serving size and limit yourself to one or two servings a day, at most, these are OK to eat.

Alcohol. Allow yourself a maximum of *one serving* per day on average.

Research shows that moderate amounts of daily alcohol (one drink daily for women, two drinks daily for men) can be beneficial to your health.[5] However, during your weight-loss program, alcohol should be limited, as it contains large amounts of "empty calories," or calories without nutrients. Alcohol also often negatively affects food choices by lowering eating inhibitions. For the best possible weight loss, limit yourself to one serving of alcohol per day at most. This may be more challenging for some due to lifestyle factors or personal preferences. If this is the case for you, while not the best choice, you may allow yourself a maximum of seven drinks per week and distribute them as you choose. I do, however, discourage drinking three to four drinks a night on weekends only, as this type of "binge" drinking can be detrimental to your health. In addition, if you are having a cocktail, opt for club soda or diet soda as a mixer, not fruit juice, tonic water, or margarita mix. These are all very high in sugar and add hundreds of calories (amounts are listed below). Consider flavored vodkas with club soda as a tasty, lower-calorie option.

CALORIES IN COMMON COCKTAILS

(taken from *The Doctor's Pocket Calorie Fat & Carb Counter* by Allan Borushek (Costa Mesa, CA: Family Health Publications, 2001), 149–154)

Beer—light (12 oz.)	95–110
Beer—regular (12 oz.)	125–165
Bloody Mary	95
Cordial (1 oz.)—Baileys, Kahlua, Schnapps, Amaretto	95–105
Cosmopolitan	215
Champagne (4 oz.)	85
Daiquiri (4 oz.)	265
Eggnog	270
Gin and Tonic	220
Irish Coffee	175
Long Island Tea	290
Mai Tai	220
Margarita (6 oz.)	180
Martini	135
Mojito	160

Piña Colada	325
Screwdriver	160
Tom Collins	210
Vodka, Rum, Tequila, Whiskey, Gin (1 oz.)	65
White Russian (6 oz.)	410
Whiskey Sour	150

Fruits. Aim for *two to three servings* per day.

Fruits are a good source of fiber, are relatively low in calories, and are chock-full of vitamins, minerals, and phytonutrients. This does not mean that you can eat unlimited amounts of all types of fruit if your goal is weight loss. Fruits higher in naturally occurring fruit sugar can still impact your blood sugar and make you feel hungrier sooner. Also, while fruits are lower in calories than most foods, they still have calories, which can add up if you're not monitoring the number of servings and portion sizes. Women frequently make this common mistake, not even counting the fruit calories in their daily diet. I'm not suggesting that fruit is unhealthy, but I have a few suggestions to optimize your fruit intake for weight loss.

Limit fruit juice. Fruit juice does not contain fiber, which is important for fullness and weight loss. Juice is also a concentrated form of calories and can be quickly consumed. Think about the amount of time that it takes you to eat an orange versus the amount of time it takes to drink a four-ounce glass of juice. If you can't live without juice, have a small (four-ounce) glass in the morning with your protein-based breakfast, but get rid of the jumbo juice goblet for good.

Do not eat higher-sugar fruit alone. For maximum hunger and blood sugar control, try to eat most fruit, especially higher-sugar or higher-carbohydrate fruits, with a little lean protein or healthy fat. This will help keep blood sugar and hunger levels under control. If you are having trouble losing weight or have high normal blood sugar or diabetes, you may consider cutting higher-sugar fruits for a time. I have found that peri- and postmenopausal women may also be more sensitive to the effects of high-sugar fruits. Most lower-sugar fruits can be eaten alone, but if you find that you get hungry shortly after eating a low-sugar fruit, combine it with lean protein or fat to fill you up longer.

Stay away from dried fruit. Unlike juice, dried fruit contains fiber, but it does not contain water, so dried fruit is a much more concentrated source of calories and can add up quickly. Imagine how quickly you could eat ten dried apricots versus ten whole apricots, or two tablespoons of raisins versus two cups of grapes. Besides, whole fruit is much more filling. So stick with the whole fruit, save calories, *and* feel fuller!

Fruit Serving Sizes
Lower sugar
  Apple: 1 small, fresh
  Blueberries: ¾ cup
  Cantaloupe: 1 cup, freshly diced
  Cherries (3 oz.): 12 fresh cherries
  Grapefruit: ½, fresh
  Kiwi: 1, fresh
  Orange: 1 small, fresh
  Peach: 1 medium, fresh

Pear: ½ large, fresh

Plum: 2 medium

Raspberries: 1 cup, fresh

Strawberries: 1 ¼ cup (12 large whole), fresh or 1 cup, frozen

Watermelon: 1 slice (13 ½ oz.) or 1 ¼ cup, freshly cubed

Higher sugar

Apricots: 6 dried halves or ½ cup, canned

Banana (4 oz.): ½ large or 1 small

Grapes: ¾ cup

Mango: ½ cup

Papaya: ½ cup

Pineapple: ¾ cup, freshly diced

Raisins: 2 tablespoons

Vegetables. Eat a minimum of *five servings* daily (fresh or frozen are best). Serving size = ½ cup cooked or juice or 1 cup raw = 25 calories. Total Daily Goal = 2 ½ cups cooked or 5 cups raw (or any combination of cooked and raw vegetables).

The majority of Americans do not eat enough vegetables (unless you count french fries and catsup). Here are a few probable reasons:

1. Most vegetables are not as portable and convenient as other foods.
2. Most vegetables take longer to prepare than other foods.
3. Most vegetables don't taste as good alone as other foods.

Along with most nutrition experts, I strongly believe that increasing your vegetable consumption is one of the keys to successful long-term weight loss. My goal in this book is to try to make increasing your vegetable intake as easy as possible by showing you ways of making vegetables simpler, tastier, and more convenient. Since I don't know how to cook, you can rest assured that none of my suggestions will require a lot of time. Check out the recipes and shopping list sections at the end of the book for lots of ideas on quick, easy, and tasty veggie recipes.

It is important that you put a little effort into vegetable variety and making vegetables taste good. This will not only ensure that you get all the nutrients you need, but will also prevent diet boredom. Research shows that successful dieters have more variety in their vegetable consumption and eat significantly more vegetables when they are prepared with more flavor.[6,7] Aspire to try a new vegetable serving suggestion, recipe, or restaurant dish on a regular basis.

Though there is no such thing as an unhealthy vegetable, there are several vegetable superstars listed in the Top 10 Veggies chart that follows. In particular, dark green and colorful orange and red vegetables pack an extra health punch. By incorporating some of these into your diet on a regular basis, you will not only be slimmer but much healthier too. And for those of you who insist that you don't like any vegetables (I have several patients who have sheepishly admitted this to me), here's a complete list for you to review. I hope you find at least five vegetables that, with the right preparation, you can routinely incorporate into your diet:

Top 10 Veggies

Swiss chard	Spinach
Kale	Brussels sprouts

Broccoli	Carrots
Sweet potato (starch)	Butternut squash (starch)
Red bell pepper	Asparagus

The Rest of the Bunch
(Check off your favorites as a reminder to incorporate them into your diet.)

❑ Artichoke	❑ Onions
❑ Artichoke hearts	❑ Parsnips
❑ Bean sprouts	❑ Pea pods
❑ Beets	❑ Peppers
❑ Cabbage	❑ Radishes
❑ Cauliflower	❑ Salad greens (endive,
❑ Celery	escarole, lettuce,
❑ Cucumber	romaine)
❑ Eggplant	❑ Summer squash
❑ Green beans	❑ Tomato
❑ Green onions	❑ Tomato sauce
❑ Green bell pepper	❑ Turnip greens
❑ Leeks	❑ Turnips
❑ Mushrooms	❑ Water chestnuts
❑ Mustard greens	❑ Watercress
❑ Okra	❑ Zucchini

Fats. 5 grams of fat = 45 calories. *Women* should aim for *four to six servings* per day depending on their size. *Men* should get *five to seven servings* per day depending on size.

As with protein intake, smaller, lighter people should stay on the lower end of the range; larger, heavier people can stay toward the higher end. It may be necessary to adjust your intake as you lose weight, since you will require fewer calories.

Not all fat is bad for your health. In fact, there are several types of healthy fats, and even some "super fats" that help prevent and treat disease and may actually improve your health. Without some fat in your diet, you can suffer from vitamin deficiencies, dry skin, a drop in good cholesterol, and suboptimal health. However, for weight loss, it is important to recognize that fat has more than double the calories per gram of either protein or carbohydrates. It is therefore critical to watch your serving sizes of fat closely, as fat calories add up more quickly than any other kind. You should not, however, cut fat completely from your diet. Healthy fats cannot only boost health, but they make food more enjoyable and can help keep you fuller longer, thereby enhancing weight loss.

SUPER FATS

The healthiest fats are the omega-3 fatty acids. These "super" fats can lessen your risk of sudden death from a heart attack; help lower triglycerides; cut stroke risk; may decrease risk of breast, endometrial, and prostate cancer; aid treatment of rheumatoid arthritis; and even play a role in the treatment of depression and Alzheimer's.[8] Omega-3 fatty acids are so important to heart health that for the first time in its history the American Heart Association has endorsed taking fish oil supplements. Try to get 500–1,000 mg a day of omega-3 fats. Talk to your doctor about taking more than this amount if you have specific health concerns. See options for optimizing omega-3 intake below.

Consume omega-3–rich seafood at least twice a week. Top sources include salmon, trout, sardines, herring, oysters, mackerel, sole, halibut, cod, and tuna, but most other seafood and shellfish contain some too. (Note that frying fish negates the beneficial effects of omega-3 fats.)

If you prefer to take fish oil capsules, most contain 180 mg EPA and 120 mg DHA. Take one to three capsules daily with food. Side effects can include belching. To avoid this, look for enteric-coated capsules. A recent study by Consumer Lab, an independent testing group, found no contaminants (like PCBs) among forty-one fish oil supplements that they tested, which is good news for consumers. (To obtain this report, please go to www.consumerlab.com/results/omega3.asp.)

If you don't eat fish and don't like the idea of taking fish oil capsules, try eating foods rich in ALA, a plant-based omega-3 fatty acid, some of which can be converted to EPA and DHA by the body. Good sources include walnuts, soybeans, ground or whole flaxseed or flaxseed oil, and canola oil.

Fat Serving Sizes

Healthy fats (these fats in small quantities should represent most of your daily fat intake):

1 teaspoon canola, extra virgin olive oil, or flaxseed oil

¼ avocado

Olives: 8 large black, 10 large green

Nuts/seeds(⅛ cup = 1 Fat, ½ Protein): almonds,
  cashews, peanuts, pecans, walnuts, sunflower seeds,
  pumpkin seeds
Nut butters: 1 tablespoon = 1 Fat, ½ Protein

Less healthy fats (these fats should be somewhat limited):
  1 teaspoon margarine or 1 tablespoon light margarine
  1 teaspoon mayo or 1 tablespoon light mayo
  1 teaspoon corn, safflower, soybean oil
  Non-olive- or canola-oil-based salad dressing:
    1 tablespoon regular, 2 tablespoons low-fat

Saturated fats (these fats should be very limited):
  1 teaspoon butter (stick, tub, or liquid) or 1 tablespoon
    reduced-fat or light butter
  1 tablespoon (½ oz.) cream cheese or 2 tablespoons (1 oz.)
    reduced-fat or light cream cheese
  2 tablespoons of sour cream or 3 tablespoons of reduced-
    fat or light sour cream
  2 tablespoons of half-and-half cream or nondairy liquid
    coffee whitener
  1 slice of cooked bacon
  1 tablespoon cream-based salad dressing

Trans Fats. These fats are one of the real nutrition vil-
lains. They start out as healthy fats, but through processing
designed to increase their shelf life, they are transformed
into the most deadly type of fat for your heart. Trans fats are
present in many foods, including vegetable shortening, margarines, baked goods, snack foods, fried foods, and many

processed foods. Not only do they raise bad cholesterol, but they also lower good cholesterol. This lethal combination is up to two times worse for your heart health than saturated fat. Beginning in 2006, the FDA required companies to list the amount of trans fats on labels, but if a product has less than 0.5 grams of trans fats, the product can be categorized as "trans fat free." Since there is no safe level of trans fats, and health organizations recommend consuming no more than 2 grams per day of trans fats, it is important to look at food labels for the word *hydrogenated* (or *partially hydro-genated*). Try to limit your consumption of products with these types of fats. At the very least, make sure that they are very low on the list of ingredients. The good news is that, due to increased public awareness, companies are working hard to remove these deadly fats from their products.

Reading Labels

Understanding how to read labels is an important component of enduring success if you eat packaged foods frequently. Do not spend too much time trying to figure out exactly how to classify everything you eat, but do try to understand what you are eating. More importantly, compare labels of similar foods so that you can make the best possible choices. To figure out how packaged food translates into specific food groups, use this table.

| 1 Starch | 80 calories | 15 g. carbohydrates, 3 g. protein, 0–1 g. fat |

1 Low-fat Protein	40 calories	7 g. protein, up to 1.5 g. fat
1 Fat	45 calories	5 g. fat
1 Fruit	60 calories	15 g. carbohydrates
1 Vegetable	25 calories	5 g. carbohydrates
1 Dairy	90 calories	8 g. protein, 12 g. carbohydrates

When looking at food labels, you must keep in mind the type of food you are eating. If you see 12 grams of sugar in one yogurt cup and 35 grams in another, this suggests that the 35-gram cup has 23 grams of added sugar—almost 6 extra teaspoons. If you are going to eat 23 grams of sugar, I'd rather you have it in the form of an actual treat, like chocolate or a cookie, not yogurt. If you see one box of cereal with 33 grams of carbohydrates and 13 grams of sugar, and another box also has 33 grams of carbohydrates but 22 grams of sugar, the first box is obviously the healthier option, though both are slightly higher in carbs.

There are no strict rules on what to look for when reading labels, so consider the entire label, not just fat content, calories, or sugar grams. If a food is very low in sugar but very high in saturated fat, it is not a great choice. If a food is very low in calories but very high in sugar, again, it is not the best choice. Here are a few tips to help steer you toward healthier products.

Label Reading 101

Serving size. Ignorance of the actual serving size is one of the most common nutrition mistakes that I see, especially with products that appear to be a single serving. Pay close attention both to the serving size *and* the servings per container. Many food makers try to make their products seem healthier or lower in calories by listing a serving size that is often not the amount you actually consume. For example, my favorite healthy muffins list the serving size as ½ muffin. They are very healthy and low in calories, but I doubt that most people eat half a muffin. My favorite all-natural soy protein snack chips (Kay's) come in a bag that appears to be single serving size, but the full bag *really* contains 1.4 servings. They are still healthy, but when you consider how quickly an extra 50 calories can add up here and there, it is important to be aware of how much you are actually consuming.

Ingredients list. I am fairly certain that most people don't even look at the ingredient list on food labels, which is unfortunate. This part of the label is very informative. Ingredients are listed in the order of their amounts in that product. For example, if sugar or high-fructose corn syrup is listed toward the top of the ingredient list, assume that there is a lot of added sugar in that particular product. If you see the words *whole grain* at the top of a list, the product contains less processed carbohydrates. In general, the more ingredients that you don't recognize or cannot pronounce, the more highly processed the food. Do your best to avoid foods with partially hydrogenated oils near the top of the ingredient list, and minimize foods with these toxic trans fats anywhere in the ingredients list.

Carbohydrates. Under this heading, both sugar and fiber will be listed. Rather than give you strict rules, I would prefer that you compare similar products and always try to choose the lower-sugar, higher-fiber goods. Remember that grains are one of the best sources of fiber, so try to choose bread with at least two grams of fiber per slice and cereals with at least five grams of fiber per serving. When figuring out the number of starch servings in a packaged food, fiber and sugar alcohols are subtracted from the total carbohydrate count since they are minimally absorbed by the body. Don't forget that dairy products have twelve grams of carbohydrates per serving, but they are not considered a starch. The carbohydrates are from milk sugar, which is different from starchy carbohydrates. Also, vegetables contain five grams of carbohydrates per serving, so if a frozen dinner or soup contains a lot of veggies, this would count as a vegetable serving, not a starch. Try not to overanalyze the label; just pay attention to what you are actually eating.

Fat. Total fat, saturated fat, and trans fat will all be listed. Try to minimize both saturated and trans fats. The remaining fat is not necessarily unhealthy, but remember that all fat calories add up more quickly than protein or carbohydrates, so try to limit the total fat in packaged foods. Of course, nuts and oil-based foods are *made up* of fat, so it is impossible to limit the fat content in these foods. Here you must just watch your serving sizes.

Percent Daily Values. I don't recommend paying too much attention to percent daily values, because for most nutrients they are too general to be useful. You should pay some attention to the sodium (salt) values, especially if you have high blood pressure, and to the calcium values if you are a woman and are not taking a calcium supplement. Most packaged foods have high sodium levels, so compare labels and try to choose lower-sodium options when available. And don't forget to note the serving size when calculating sodium content to determine how much salt you are actually eating.

Look at the practice label on the next page.

At this point, you should feel confident that you have the basic nutrition knowledge about food groups and understand the approximate quantities of each food group that you should personally consume daily for optimal weight loss. Now let's put this knowledge into action with realistic meal ideas and options that even the busiest person can work into his or her schedule.

Nutrition Facts	
Serving Size	1 Cup (53g/1.9 oz.)
Servings Per Container	About 23

Amount Per Serving	Cereal
Calories	190
Calories from Fat	25
	Percent Daily Value **
Total Fat 3g 5 percent	
Saturated Fat 0g	0 percent
Trans Fat 0g	0 percent
Cholesterol 0mg	0 percent
Sodium 95mg	4 percent
Potassium 300mg	9 percent
Total Carbohydrate 36g	12 percent
Dietary Fiber 8g	32 percent
Soluble Fiber 3g	
Insoluble Fiber 5g	
Sugars 13g	
Other Carbohydrate 15g	
Protein 9g	14 percent
Vitamin A	0 percent
Vitamin C	0 percent
Calcium	4 percent
Iron	10 percent
Phosporus	10 percent
Magnesium	10 percent
Copper	8 percent

**Percent Daily Values are based on a 2,000 calorie diet. Your daily values may be higher or lower depending on your calorie needs.

Ingredients: Kashi® Seven Whole Grains & Sesame Cereal (Whole: oats, long grain brown rice, barley, sesame seeds), textured soy protein concentrate, evaporated cane juice, brown rice syrup, chicory root fiber (inulin), whole grain oats, Kashi® Seven Whole Grains Sesame Flour (Whole: oats, long grain brown rice, rye, hard red winter wheat, triticale, buckwheat, barley, sesame seeds), expeller pressed canola oil, honey, salt, cinnamon, mixed tocopherols (natural vitamin E) for freshness.

This cereal is slightly higher in calories per serving but a great source of fiber and a good source of protein, so very satisfying.

Great source of both types of fiber. After subtracting fiber, this would count as 2 starches (15 grams of carbohydrate per starch)

This is good example of a healthy ingredients list. No hydrogenated oils, lots of whole grains, all-natural sugars, no preservatives.

THREE

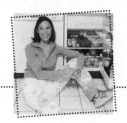

The Busy Person's Meal Ideas

Many of my patients are a bit overwhelmed with nutrition knowledge at this point and just want to know what to eat. Before I go into specific meal ideas, I want to give you an overview of what your day should look like. There is no "one way to eat" that works for everyone. By understanding the big picture outlined in the Sample Menu Day section, you can really build a weight-loss program into your life rather than turning your life upside down to lose weight.

SAMPLE MENU DAY

This is an outline of what your day should look like. It is not necessarily meant to be followed exactly but to give you an overview of what kinds of things you can eat at different meals and snacks. Customize this eating plan to your own lifestyle and eating patterns (but don't sacrifice the basic principles). If you don't get very hungry in the morning, have a light breakfast and a larger morning snack. If you eat breakfast at eight and lunch at noon, and you find that you don't get hungry in between or arrive at lunch famished, skip the morning snack or integrate the morning snack into breakfast or lunch. If you get hungry a few hours after dinner, cut back a little at an earlier meal or snack and add a nighttime snack. Just remember to follow the basic points below:

- Try to have some form of protein (or dairy) with every meal and snack.
- Minimize starches at night.
- Watch serving sizes of fats (including high-fat protein) and starches the most.

Breakfast
0–2 starches
   or 1 starch + 1 fruit
2–3 proteins and/or 1 dairy
1–2 fats (optional)

Snack (optional)
1–2 proteins or 1 dairy
1 fruit or starch
1 fat (optional)

Lunch
0–2 starches
3–4 proteins
1–2 veggies
1–2 fats (optional)

Snack
1–2 proteins or 1 dairy
1 fruit or starch
1 fat (optional)

Dinner
4–6 lean proteins
0–2 starches (limit)
2–3 veggies
1–2 fats (optional)

Snack (optional)
1–2 proteins or 1 dairy
1 fruit
1 fat (optional)

THE BUSY PERSON'S BREAKFAST IDEAS AND OPTIONS

You do not have to limit yourself to this list of meals. Feel free to invent your own meals using the Sample Menu Day outline. Women, in general, should eat the smaller serving sizes listed. If you are not a breakfast person, you don't have to eat a lot, but you must have something in the morning, even if it is just a protein bar. Research consistently shows that people who eat breakfast are more successful (both in the short run and the long run) with weight loss.[1] Eating breakfast may also improve insulin sensitivity and help you eat less throughout the day.[2] (And don't forget to count your morning latte; it has calories too.)

Yogurt and Fruit Crunch (This is my patients' favorite breakfast choice!)
1 cup plain or low-sugar yogurt (Fage's Total Greek yogurt, Dannon Light 'n Fit, Yoplait Light/Ultra)
¼ to ½ cup berries (fresh or frozen)
¼ to ½ cup low-fat granola or high-fiber cereal (Kashi GoLean Crunch! is my favorite)
On-the-go option: Bring yogurt, an apple, and cereal (prepacked in a zip-lock bag).

PB & J sandwich

1–2 slices whole-grain toast or a whole wheat English muffin

1–2 tablespoons all-natural peanut butter (organic peanut butter is best) and 1–2 teaspoons low-sugar jelly

On-the-go option: Bring a sandwich to your favorite coffee spot and enjoy with a small nonfat latte instead of the usual muffin or pastry.

Edgy Omelet

3-egg-white omelet or 1 full egg plus 2 whites or ½ cup egg substitute

½ cup to 1 cup fresh or frozen vegetables (spinach, onions, mushrooms, etc.)

(Optional) Top with 2 tablespoons low-fat cheddar cheese or 1 tablespoon fresh grated Parmesan

1–2 slices of whole-grain toast with 1 teaspoon butter

EGG-CELLENT NEWS

A 1996 article by medical writer Kathleen Meister, titled "Eggs: Not as Bad as They're Cracked Up to Be" (*Priorities* 8, no. 3), dispels the myth that eggs are "bad for you." (You can read the complete article on the American Council on Science and Health Web site at www.acsh.org/publications/pubID.716/pub_detail.asp.) For most people, the cholesterol in egg yolks will not have a substantial effect on their cholesterol levels. Saturated fat has a much more significant effect.

Eggs are inexpensive and easy to prepare, and egg whites are made of some of the highest quality protein available. Egg yolks also contain important nutrients, like choline and lutein. In one research study, people who ate eggs for breakfast instead of a bagel felt less hungry before lunch, and ate less both at lunch and throughout the entire day.[3] Of course, don't forget that egg yolks have two-and-a-half times the calories of egg whites, so I recommend limiting yourself to one whole egg and adding egg whites for extra protein. (If you have high bad cholesterol, you may want to stick solely with egg whites, just to be safe.)

Dr. Melina's Homemade Breakfast Sandwich

1 egg or 2 whites or ¼ cup Egg Beaters, scrambled (or slice a hard-boiled egg in half)
1 low-fat vegetarian sausage patty (Morningstar), slice of ham, or low-fat cheese
Whole-grain English muffin (half or whole muffin)

Power Oatmeal

½ to 1 cup cooked plain/nonsweetened or low-sugar oatmeal (add Splenda and cinnamon for flavor)
1 scoop of plain or vanilla protein powder (use a bit more water than recipe says) or ½ cup cottage cheese
(Optional) ¼ to ½ cup berries

On-the-go and travel option: Instant oatmeal packet (with or without added protein), hard-boiled egg, 1 serving fruit

Cottage Cheese and Fruit

½ to ¾ cup cottage cheese plus ¼ to ½ cup berries (fresh or frozen)

(Optional)1 slice whole-grain toast with 2 teaspoons peanut butter

On-the-go option: Knudsen's cottage cheese singles (or doubles with fruit), 1 serving fruit, high-fiber cereal bar (optional)

Protein Smoothie

Mix 1 scoop of vanilla protein powder with 1 cup of nonfat milk or water and ½ to 1 cup fresh or frozen berries. Add Splenda to taste (or try chocolate protein powder with ½ banana and 1 tablespoon peanut butter)

(Optional) 1 slice whole-grain toast with 2 teaspoons peanut butter

On-the-go option: Yogurt smoothie (low sugar) or protein drink (EAS carb control) plus All-Bran high-fiber cereal bar (or other high-fiber granola bar)

Quick and Tasty Quiche Cups (See recipe in Appendix B.)
Also a good on-the-go option with a piece of fruit.

Fast Frittata (See recipe in Appendix B.)

Apple "Danish" (See recipe in Appendix B.)
Also makes a tasty dessert.

Super Cereal (serving sizes vary by cereal)

¾ cup (or 1 ½ cup) high-fiber cereal, like Kashi GoLean, with 1 cup nonfat milk. Note, you may want to add ½ scoop of plain or vanilla protein powder to your milk prior to pouring over cereal for a little extra protein.

If you find that you are very hungry one to two hours after eating cereal, skip this Super Cereal option.

Breakfast Burrito

1 egg and 2 whites or ½ cup Egg Beaters scrambled with ¼ cup of salsa or veggies (onions, peppers), topped with (Optional) 1 slice low-fat cheese, served in 1–2 small low-carb tortillas

Better Than Nothing

Nonfat latte protein bar (See chart in Appendix A for suggestions, or go to my Web site, www.drmelina.com, to purchase the nutrition bar that I designed.)

THE BUSY PERSON'S LUNCH IDEAS AND OPTIONS

If you are like most of my patients, you probably have no time to prepare your lunch or to sit down to a lengthy meal. The lunch options listed below are for those who are motivated enough to cook or at least put together a quick lunch. For the majority of you who prefer to eat out, I have included a few options here, but please review the section on dining out for a full range of choices. You are usually safe with a large salad with protein, as long as you watch the toppings, or a sandwich on whole wheat bread with lean protein. There are also several great premade salads at stores like Trader Joe's and Whole Foods as well as numerous preprepared meals on the shopping lists in Appendix D.

SANDWICH SURPRISES

Tuna salad, egg salad, and chicken salad sandwiches may seem healthy, but because of the mayonnaise, they can have the same amount of calories as a Philly cheesesteak. So keep it simple—skip the cheese, mayo, and any other special sauce, and save hundreds of calories. And don't be fooled by the healthy "vegetarian" option. It usually comes with avocado and cheese and can have more than double the calories of a turkey sandwich with mustard.

Pita Pocket
½ whole wheat pita
Stuff with 2–3 ounces protein (chicken, lean ham
    or roast beef, turkey, tuna).
Add 2 tablespoons hummus, guacamole, tzaziki,
    or salsa.
Add ½ cup vegetables if available (lettuce, tomato,
    fresh spinach).
1 serving soy pretzels or soy chips or apple

Tuna Melt

Whole wheat English muffin (half or whole muffin)

Top with a small can or half of a large can of tuna packed in water (drain first).

Add 1 slice low-fat cheese, and heat in microwave or toaster.

1 cup grapes or berries for dessert

Turkey Roll Up

Spread 1–2 low-carb tortillas with Dijon mustard, hummus, or any low-fat dip or spread.

Add 1–2 ounces sliced turkey and ½ cup fresh spinach, and roll into a wrap.

Dannon Light 'n Fit vanilla yogurt for dessert

Cottage Cheese and Soup

½ cup to 1 cup cottage cheese

4 Ak-Mak crackers (optional)

1 cup soup: lentil (skip the crackers), chicken and vegetable, chicken and barley (skip the crackers), minestrone, butternut squash, or onion

SALAD DO'S AND DON'TS

Salads are a very satisfying and healthy lunch choice, but they are also a source of hidden calories. Typical salad toppings can easily add hundreds of calories. When making your own salad, you don't have to cut these toppings completely, but choose just a few, in smaller quantities. If you are buying premade salads, remove some of the higher-calorie toppings.

Bacon bits: 1 ounce = 150 calories
Croutons: 1 ounce = 130 calories
Raisins: 2 tablespoons = 90 calories
Shredded cheese: 1 ounce = 114 calories
Sunflower seeds or nuts: 2 tablespoons = 90 calories

Dressing Details. An average restaurant serving is probably at least $\frac{1}{4}$ cup (4 tablespoons), and the "light" version is not calorie free; it is generally about half the calories of the regular version.

Balsamic vinaigrette: $\frac{1}{4}$ cup = 180 calories
Blue Cheese: $\frac{1}{4}$ cup = 300 calories
Caesar: $\frac{1}{4}$ cup = 280 calories
French/Italian: $\frac{1}{4}$ cup = 240 calories
Ranch: $\frac{1}{4}$ cup = 360 calories
Thousand Island: $\frac{1}{4}$ cup = 260 calories

Salad dressing is one of the leading sources of fat in the American diet and is a very frequent source of hidden calories. In my practice, salad dressing is often one of the explanations for patients not losing weight. Consider the following story.

A few years ago, I had a patient who worked in the legal profession, and he loved to argue with me about everything. He had been coming to me for a few months when, for no apparent reason, his weight loss stopped. He insisted that he was doing exactly what I told him to do, but on reviewing his food journal, I noticed that he did not specify the amount of olive oil–based dressing that he was putting on his salads at lunch. I explained that even though olive oil is very healthy, too much could interfere with weight loss. He felt that this was not the problem but agreed to cut back to one tablespoon of olive oil. To his surprise, he came in the next week with a three-pound weight loss. Don't make this mistake too. Get regular salad dressing on the side, and dip your fork in it before every bite. Or squeeze fresh lemon juice or vinegar on salads, and skip the oil if you prefer.

Low-fat Chicken Quesadilla
1–2 low-carb tortillas
1 ounce reduced-fat cheese or 1–2 tablespoons guacamole
2 ounces chicken
¼ to ½ cup salsa or chopped tomatoes
(Optional) Add a few tablespoons of fat-free refried beans for extra fiber.

Turkey or Vegetarian Chili
1–1 ½ cups low-fat or vegetarian turkey chili
Side salad or bag of carrots

Healthy Spaghetti and Meatballs
½ cup to 1 cup whole wheat pasta
3 Trader Joe's or frozen turkey meatballs
¼ cup marinara sauce

Add veggies to the mix for optimal health (cooked broccoli, cauliflower, zucchini) or have a side salad.

THE BUSY PERSON'S SNACK IDEAS AND OPTIONS

Remember that including some form of protein with most snacks is the key to minimizing hunger, maximizing metabolism, and keeping blood sugar and energy levels at their best. The only exceptions are low-sugar, high-fiber fruits (especially apples) and nonstarchy vegetables, which can be eaten alone or with low-fat dip anytime you are hungry. I strongly suggest that you always try to include protein with your afternoon snack. Finally, do not double up on fats for snacks (for example, don't eat nuts and cheese together). Try to always include a lower energy-density food like a fruit, vegetable, or dairy if you are having a high-fat food like cheese or nuts to fill you up without overdoing the number of calories.

- ⅛ to ¼ cup of nuts plus apple (OK to eat either alone if you are not very hungry)
- ½ cup cottage cheese plus ½ cup berries (Knudsen's On-the-Go with fruit is an easy option)
- String cheese and fruit (OK to eat either alone)
- Celery sticks or apple with 1–2 tablespoons of peanut butter
- 14 baby carrots or 1 cup snap peas plus 2 tablespoons hummus
- Cheese and crackers: 2–4 Ak-Mak crackers plus 1–2 ounces low-fat cheese (for easy portion control, try Mini Babybel Light cheese or Laughing Cow cheese spread)

- Yogurt cup: 1 cup plain or low-sugar yogurt alone or with 1–2 tablespoons chopped nuts, low-fat granola, or high-fiber cereal
- Protein bar or protein drink: Try to choose lower-sugar, higher-protein options (high fiber is a bonus). See the protein bar list in Appendix A for more information on selecting healthier protein bars. I developed my own line of nutrition bars that are exactly to my specifications. They are a great source of protein and fiber and are perfect for snacks. See my Web site, www.drmelina.com, for more information. Another interesting product, LightFull Satiety Smoothie, has both lean protein and is a very good source of fiber and, therefore, may be useful as a weight-loss snack.
- Quick Quesadilla: Whole wheat, low-carb tortilla with a slice of low-fat cheese (melted optional) and 2 tablespoons salsa
- Cheese Roll: Wrap low-fat or regular string cheese in whole wheat, low-carb tortilla or spread a light cheese spread on a low-carb tortilla and roll up.
- Healthy Peanut Butter Roll: Spread whole wheat, low-carb tortilla with 1 tablespoon of peanut butter and 5–10 chocolate chips.

THE BUSY PERSON'S DINNER IDEAS AND OPTIONS

While you certainly don't have to eat a three-course meal for dinner, the quick and easy suggestions below demonstrate that you can, even with restricted starchy carbohydrates, limited time, and no cooking ability! These meal ideas are not really meant for someone who likes to spend time cooking, so if you love to cook, just use these ideas as guidelines. One of the most important aspects of having a satisfying dinner without a lot of starch is to really try to make the food you eat taste good, with minimal effort, of course. Since most of my busy patients eat out frequently, and since I don't personally cook, these dinner suggestions include very simple recipes, heat-and-eat options, or suggestions for dining out or ordering in. For those of you who do love the kitchen, feel free to follow any lower-fat, lower-carbohydrate, lean-protein, and vegetable-based recipe.

Appetizers

Option 1: Salad with dressing on the side (Watch cheese and nut toppings because they add up quickly.)

Option 2: 1 cup low-fat vegetable soup (minestrone, butternut squash, low-sodium tomato, or mushroom)

Option 3: Precut raw veggies (carrots, radishes, broccoli, snap peas, cauliflower, cherry tomatoes) with premade or quick and easy low-fat dip or dressing (See appendices for recipes and shopping lists.)

Option 4: Shrimp cocktail or ceviche (raw fish salad)

Entrées

Tasty Stir-Fry. (See Appendix B for recipe or get frozen mix.) (Optional) Serve with ½ to 1 cup of brown rice if you have not exceeded your daily starch.

Quick and Easy Entrée Salad. (See recipe ideas in Appendix B or get prepackaged salads at Whole Foods, Trader Joe's, or

any grocery store.) Make sure the salad includes at least 3
ounces of lean protein. If protein and vegetables alone do
not fill you up, add a small serving of beans for extra fiber.

Protein and Vegetables. Buy precooked 3–6 ounce servings
of lean protein (chicken, salmon, tuna steak, lean pork,
turkey). Serve with a large side of any of the tasty
vegetable recipes listed in Appendix B.

Easy Chicken Chili. (See Appendix B for recipe or use canned
chicken chili and add a can of chopped tomatoes to
"dilute" the calories and lower the energy density.)

Easy Mexican Wrap. (See Appendix B for recipe or get takeout burrito without rice, throw out the tortilla, and
place the filling in a bowl or transfer filling to 1–2 whole
wheat low-carbohydrate tortillas.)

2-Minute Tortilla Soup. (See Appendix B for recipe.)

Desserts (choose 1)

- Healthy Choice Premium Fudge Bar
- Sugar-free hot chocolate
- Sugar-free, fat-free instant pudding (premade)
- ½ cup blueberries (fresh or frozen) topped with 2
  tablespoons fat-free Cool Whip
- Sugar-free Jell-O topped with 1–2 tablespoons of fat-free
  Cool Whip
- ½ to 1 cup Greek yogurt with 1 teaspoon vanilla
  extract or ½ teaspoon cinnamon and 1 packet
  of Splenda (This is my absolute favorite dessert.
  I have it almost every night!!)
- ½ to 1 cup strawberries dipped in ¼ cup
  vanilla yogurt

- 2–3 Droste dark chocolate pastilles
- Apple "Danish" (See Appendix B for recipe.)

SUPPLEMENTING YOUR DIET

While I strongly believe that food is the best source of vitamins and minerals, eating a complete and balanced diet every day is challenging, especially if you are cutting calories to lose weight. For this reason, I am a firm believer in taking a complete daily multivitamin. Choosing one, however, can be tricky, since the vitamin industry is not directly regulated by the Food and Drug Administration (FDA). In general, try to choose a reputable company that makes products according to GMP (good manufacturing practice) standards.

You do not have to spend a fortune for good quality vitamins, and it is not necessary to take a product with twenty times the recommended daily amount of vitamins and minerals. Very high doses of vitamins have not been shown to be more beneficial, and some can actually be harmful. Nonetheless, be aware that the Percent Daily Values have not been updated since the 1970s and are a bit out of date. In addition, they were established to prevent nutrient deficiencies, not necessarily to achieve your best state of health. Still, if you eat a balanced diet with lots of fresh fruits and vegetables and take a basic multivitamin, you will more than likely obtain plenty of the most important vitamins and minerals—with a few exceptions described below. Finally, do not be tempted to choose specific vitamins and minerals that you may have read about for certain health benefits. Taking too much of any single nutrient can throw off your body's balance and may even cause you to be less healthy in some cases.

In addition to a complete daily multivitamin, I put almost all of my patients on a fish oil supplement. Don't worry; you don't have to drink cod-liver oil like your grandmother did, and I don't own stock in any fish oil companies. There are just so many health benefits associated with omega-3 fatty acids, and since it is a bit more challenging and expensive to get adequate amounts from diet alone, it is important to take a daily supplement for maximum health. Again, try to find a reputable company, and remember that it is not necessary to spend a fortune. The only extra feature you may want to consider paying a bit more for is enteric-coated capsules. I offer these in my office and on my Web site (www.drmelina.com) because patients do not like burping fish after ingesting non-coated supplements. I recommend 1 gram per day of fish oil (the FDA recommends a maximum of 2 grams daily). But talk with your doctor if you have a specific medical problem such as high triglycerides or arthritis that may benefit from larger doses.

I'm sorry to say that there is no magic "fat-burning" supplement. There are a few that may produce a small amount of increased fat loss, but it is usually no more than could be achieved by eating one fewer cracker per day, so I would not waste the money.

Calcium and Vitamin D
For most people, three servings of dairy per day provide more than enough calcium. However, if you do not consume at least three servings of dairy per day or are at high risk for

osteoporosis, you should probably take a calcium supplement. Vitamin D is critical for optimal calcium absorption, so try to find a supplement that includes vitamin D, particularly if you don't spend a lot of time in the sun or are older than seventy. (You can get vitamin D through the skin by sunlight exposure, but this ability decreases as you age.) Calcium carbonate is the least expensive form of calcium and is appropriate for most people. This excludes those who take antacids or medication for ulcers or heartburn and people older than seventy. Calcium citrate is better for these people, as it does not require acid for absorption.

DAILY RECOMMENDED INTAKE

Calcium	*Vitamin D*
Age 19–50 = 1000 mg/day	Age 19–50 = 5 mcg/day
Age >50 = 1200 mg/day	Age 50–70 = 10 mcg/day
	Age >70 = 15 mcg/day

(Dietary Reference Intakes, Food and Nutrition Board, Institute of Medicine)

Chromium

Chromium plays an essential role in the function of insulin. On its own and in combination with biotin (2 mg), it helps considerably to reduce blood sugar in type 2 diabetics. In addition, a dose of 600 mcg/day has been associated with significant reductions in carbohydrate cravings, and may even help with fatigue and mood swings in some. One observational study showed a trend toward weight loss and, at the very least, less weight gain among obese people taking a chromium supplement.[4]

If you have type 2 diabetes, metabolic syndrome, high blood sugar, or intense carbohydrate cravings, consider taking 400–800 mcg of this supplement. It will not necessarily aid with weight loss, but it will help with blood sugar and insulin control, which may facilitate weight loss. Diabetics should talk with their doctor before adding this supplement.

Green Tea

In addition to being a very good antioxidant, green tea also has noteworthy cholesterol-lowering effects. Research shows that a highly concentrated green tea extract (375 mg capsules EGCG, the active ingredient) reduced cholesterol by 11 percent and bad cholesterol by 16 percent in twelve weeks. Patients saw a slight increase in good cholesterol and a slight reduction in triglycerides.[5] I recommend this supplement to all of my patients with high cholesterol, particularly those who are not willing to take the powerful cholesterol-lowering medications. There is also a small amount of research showing a minimal benefit for weight loss, but it is not definitive, and at this point I am not convinced that it plays a significant role, especially in the small doses present in most "weight-loss" supplements.

You can also opt to just drink the green tea, but you would have to consume more than five cups per day to get adequate EGCG!

Cinnamon

While cinnamon is a spice, not a supplement, I thought it was worth mentioning here for its remarkable health benefits. It has been shown to improve fasting blood sugar by up to 29 percent, decrease bad cholesterol by up to 27 percent, lower triglycerides by up to 30 percent, and reduce total cholesterol by up to 16 percent.[6] I recommend adding it to your diet whenever you can. Try sprinkling it in yogurt, oatmeal, coffee, soups, chili, or any sauce that could use a bit of spice.

A Word on Water

Most nutrition experts agree that water is important for health and weight loss. Research shows that even mild dehydration can slow metabolism and that drinking water, especially when it is cold, can temporarily increase metabolism by up to 30 percent.[7]

How much is enough? We don't really know because the answer is different for everyone. Bigger people need more water. If you exercise a lot or live in a warmer climate, you need more water because of increased water loss through sweat. Aim for at least eight glasses of water per day. If you weigh more than 200 pounds, have an extra glass. Also drink an extra glass, or two, anytime you exercise for more than thirty minutes, especially in warmer temperatures. Try to drink water throughout the day. You may even want to schedule regular "water" breaks until you get into the habit of drinking water more regularly. Feel free to be creative with water intake: drink flavored sparkling water, iced green tea with lemon, Crystal Light, or an occasional diet soda.

The Busy Person's Fast-Food and Fast-Casual Options

Since fast food represents one-third of meals eaten outside the home, no diet book would be complete without providing some healthier fast-food options. While many obesity experts blame fast food for the country's rising obesity epidemic, our hectic lifestyles and limited budgets often make fast food unavoidable. While I am in no way advocating fast food, I do realize that many people who are trying to lose weight rely on fast-food and fast-casual restaurants as an eating option, so I have provided some healthier choices. If you eat fast food regularly, make sure the rest of your diet includes lots of fresh vegetables, fruits, and whole grains.

Fast-Food General Tips

- Avoid large, jumbo, or supersize *anything*. The extra calories, sugar, salt, fat, and associated health risks are not worth saving a quarter.
- Skip the fried or breaded sandwiches. Instead choose broiled or grilled options. Grilled chicken is always a good choice.
- Hold the cheese, creamy or honey sauces, and mayo, which add hundreds of calories. Stick with mustard,

ketchup, hot sauce—even BBQ sauce in small amounts is OK.

■ Avoid regular soda and sugary juice drinks, including lemonade.

■ Stay away from high-fat breads, like croissants and biscuits, which add both calories and fat.

■ Limit yourself to one fast-food meal per day, as fast food is much higher in salt (even salads) and fat than most other types of food.

■ When ordering salads, always keep the dressing on the side and dip your fork in it. Even the low-fat version can add more than one hundred calories in some cases. And watch for high-fat or high-calorie toppings, like bacon, cheese, tortilla chips, croutons, and noodles.

Now that you know the basics about ordering at a fast-food restaurant, here are a few ideas for healthier fast-food options. (Please note that I said "healthi*er*," *not* "healthy." Try to limit your consumption of fast food as much as possible.)

The Best Fast-Food Choices by Restaurant

Burger King
Hamburger
Chicken Whopper (*no* mayo; high salt)
BK Veggie Burger (*no* mayo; eat only ½ bun and save
  1 starch)
BBQ, sweet and sour sauce (all other sauces double the
  calories or more)

Side Garden Salad (free food)

Chicken Salad (get dressing on the side; even fat free = 70 calories)

Carl's Jr.

Charbroiled BBQ Chicken Sandwich

Charbroiled Chicken Salad-to-Go

Garden Salad-to-Go: fat-free Italian or dressing on the side (free food)

Chipotle (fast-casual Mexican)

Burrito Bol is a great option (no tortilla); chicken is best, but steak is pretty good too; get black beans or pinto beans, no rice, salsa, fajita vegetables; ½ serving of guacamole is optional

Salads also good option; no cheese

Denny's

Grilled Chicken Dinner

Vegetable Beef or Chicken Noodle Soup

Garden Deluxe Salad with chicken breast, turkey, or ham

Side Garden Salad

Eggs and English muffin or Toast (dry)

Healthier sides: carrots in honey glaze, green beans with bacon, sliced tomato, cottage cheese, applesauce

Domino's Pizza

Cheese or vegetable toppings are best

Start with large salad with dressing on the side.

Ask for light cheese, and stick with thin crust.

Jack in the Box
- Chicken Fajita Pita (hold cheese)
- Southwest Chicken Pita
- Breakfast Jack
- Chicken Sandwich (no cheese; no mayo)
- Asian Chicken Salad; skip the crispy wontons
- Chicken Caesar Salad (low-fat balsamic dressing OK)
- Side Salad
- Low-fat Herb Mayo

KFC
- Caesar Salad, no dressing
- Honey BBQ Sandwich, side green beans
- Tender Roast Sandwich (get hot sauce instead of regular sauce)
- Corn on the cob (small)

McDonald's
- Hamburger
- English ,muffin and 2 scrambled eggs (with coffee or water, not juice)
- Egg McMuffin (hold the cheese)
- Fruit 'n Yogurt Parfait
- Chicken McGrill; no mayo (ask for BBQ or Hot Mustard Sauce packet instead)
- Grilled Chicken-Caesar salad with reduced-fat dressing
- Vanilla reduced fat ice cream cone (my favorite occasional treat)
- Grilled Chicken Bacon Ranch Salad (Newman's Own Low-Fat Balsamic Vinaigrette OK)

Caesar Salad with Grilled Chicken, or plain
Grilled Chicken California Cobb Salad
Side Salad

Panda Express (mall outlet Chinese food)
Black Pepper Chicken
Chicken with Mushrooms
Chicken with String Beans
Chicken with Peanuts
Beef with Broccoli or String Beans
Mixed Vegetables
Soy Sauce, Hot Mustard Sauce, Hot Sauce

Panera Bread
Lower-carb breads (i.e., Italian, pumpkin) are the better
option or whole-grain baguette or loaf
Good choice of low-fat soups, including Chicken Noodle,
Vegetarian Black Bean, Moroccan Lentil, Garden
Vegetable
Asian Sesame Chicken Salad, Grilled Chicken Caesar
Salad, and Fandango Salad with Fat-free Poppyseed,
Fat-free Raspberry dressing, or Reduced-sugar Asian
Sesame Vinaigrette)
Fresh Fruit Cup

Subway
Choose any 6-inch sandwich with 6 grams of fat (Chicken,
Roast Beef, Turkey, Veggie Delite) on a whole wheat
low-carb wrap instead of bread; skip the oil, mayo, and
cheese. (This is my favorite fast-lunch option.)

Grilled Chicken and Baby Spinach Salad
Subway Club Salad
Veggie Delite Salad
Kraft Fat-Free Italian Dressing or any other on the side
Soups (1 cup): Minestrone, Cream of Broccoli, Roasted
    Chicken Noodle (high salt)
Breakfast Sandwich on Deli Round (topless, no cheese)

Taco Bell

Order items "Fresco": salsa in place of cheese and sauce
Fiesta or Express Taco Salad without shell or red strips
Ranchero Chicken Soft Taco
Grilled Steak Taco

Wendy's

Ultimate Chicken Grill Sandwich (high salt, eat ½ bun)
Small chili without cheese (adds 70 calories)
Grilled chicken with honey mustard dressing (reduced fat)
Spring Mix Salad (Pecans OK, but count as fat)
Mandarin Chicken Salad (skip crispy noodles; almonds
    OK, but count as fat)
Side Salad or Caesar Side Salad

EATING OUT ON THE TOWN

If you are like most Americans, especially if you are reading
this book and have no time to lose, eating out is probably a
nonnegotiable part of your diet. In the past thirty years, the
numbers of meals and snacks that Americans eat away from

home has almost doubled. Statistics like this may be good for the food and restaurant industry, but they aren't as good for our health. Research shows that the increases in food eaten away from home correlate strongly with rising obesity.[8] Large, tasty, and often economical portions are just part of the attraction. Eating out also has an important social and business function. While it is easier to lose weight by not eating out, this is simply not realistic for the majority of people (including myself). So I have a compiled some easy strategies for dining out. *Bon appétit!*

REALISTIC RESTAURANT STRATEGIES

- Lean protein (grilled chicken or fish) and double veggies are usually a safe option.
- Don't drink your calories. Skip the lemonade, juice, and soda, and limit alcohol. You are already probably having more calories by eating out, so don't make things worse with less-filling liquid calories.
- Consider ordering two appetizers or an appetizer and salad as your entrée, especially if you are having a cocktail or plan on sharing a little dessert.
- Split meals, or plan (and follow through) to take half home for lunch the next day.
- Order salad dressing and all sauces on the side. Then dip your fork in them before every bite for a little flavor, with far fewer calories.
- If you can't figure out what a particular dish is made of, ask your waiter. If the waiter doesn't know, skip it. When

in doubt, it's better to play it safe and not risk sabotaging your diet.

▪ Bypass the bread (most of the time). Ask the waiter not to bring it or to take it away. If your dining partner complains, keep it on his or her side of the table.

▪ Choose your starches wisely. If you have a little bread, don't eat the rice or potato too! If you decide to have a side of pasta, skip the bread.

▪ Be rational about dessert. If you budgeted dessert into your day, and it is really special, split it with a friend. Don't waste calories on the vanilla ice cream you could have anytime or a mediocre apple tart.

▪ Nothing is totally off-limits. Just try to make the best choices you can or make up for it the next day with a little more exercise or a little less fat or starch.

▪ Go for a walk or dancing after your meal. Burn any extra calories before they have a chance to be stored away on your hips or stomach!

▪ Choose dishes with names that include words like *steamed, broiled, roasted, grilled,* and *poached* instead of *fried, crispy, breaded,* and *sautéed.*

AROUND-THE-WORLD EATING OPTIONS

Mexican
▪ Start with a cup of black bean soup or tortilla soup with light (or no) cheese.
▪ Chicken or shrimp fajitas or soft tacos with whole wheat

or corn tortillas; skip the cheese, and have a little guacamole and lots of salsa.

- Chicken taco salad. Skip the cheese; don't eat the bowl.
- Chicken burrito. Skip the rice and cheese, and add extra salsa and lettuce if possible; a small amount of guacamole is OK. Ask for a whole wheat tortilla if possible, or ditch the tortilla altogether.
- Order enchiladas with green or red sauce, not cream sauce. And stick with chicken instead of cheese or beef.
- Stay away from the chip basket. You probably can't eat "just a few."
- Skip the margarita. Most have much more than 300 calories of sugar and alcohol. If you must have a cocktail, have a beer or ask for tequila with lime juice only and club soda.

Italian

- Try not to get pasta as an entrée. Have it on the side or as a primi plate—as they do in Italy. If you have bread, skip the pasta, and vice versa.
- Start with a bowl of minestrone soup, a green salad, or tomato/mozzarella.
- Avoid breaded dishes like parmigiana; opt for marsala or marinara instead.
- Skip the fatty sauces such as alfredo, carbonara, or cream, which can add hundreds of calories. Watch the pesto too—even though it is healthier, it is not calorie free.
- Ask for a side of veggies instead of pasta if possible.

Chinese

- Start with wonton, hot and sour, or egg drop soup.
- Skip the white or fried rice; ask for brown rice.
- Ask for dry wok when possible.
- Experiment with Chinese veggies, and opt for chicken, tofu, and seafood since the red meat is generally quite fatty.
- Avoid sweet-and-sour or fried dishes.
- Watch the nuts in dishes; they can add up to ½ cup or more (350 or more calories).

Thai

- Avoid coconut and peanut sauces (or get on the side). Opt for oyster or black bean sauces instead.
- Order any entrée with veggies, or get a side of veggies.
- Stick with chicken, seafood, and tofu, all lower-fat options.
- Consider chicken/tofu/shrimp satay as an appetizer, or a cucumber salad.
- Skip the Thai tea. It's pure sugar and cream.

Japanese

- Start with miso soup, edamame (soy beans), or salad.
- Skip tempura (and any rolls with tempura).
- Sushi: 4 pieces of sushi = approximately ½ cup rice (1 starch), so limit to 8 pieces, *maximum*.
- Watch higher-fat ingredients in rolls, like cream cheese, avocado, and mayo in spicy tuna or crab; they add hundreds of calories.
- Sashimi is a great choice.

Deli Tips

- Avoid mayo-based sandwiches, like tuna salad, chicken salad, or egg salad, which contain hundreds of extra calories.
- Opt for lean meat, and consider eating sandwiches open-faced.
- Get dressing on the side of any salad.
- Skip or remove most of the cheese and bacon on Chef or Cobb Salads. Stick with the avocado and a dressing on the side.

Pizza

- Stick with mainly veggie toppings (chicken and ham/pineapple are OK too).
- Ask for light cheese if possible, or take a bit off.
- Start with a salad to tame your appetite slightly.
- Ask for whole wheat or thin crust.
- Avoid pesto pizza; it adds a lot of extra fat.

French

- Simple is better—if it sounds complicated, it is probably not good for your diet.
- Skip the sauces and preparation methods that are super high fat like crème, au gratin, au beurre, hollandaise, and more.

Steak House

- Start with shrimp cocktail or salad (dressing on side), not the crab cakes.
- Opt for leaner cuts, like filet mignon, instead of sirloin, prime rib, or porterhouse.

- If you must have the baked potato, eat only half, and limit the high-fat toppings.
- Stay away from the garlic mashed potatoes and creamed spinach.

Brunch

- Omelets are an easy choice, and you can get creative with toppings (egg white or Egg Beaters are best, but whole eggs on occasion are OK; just skip the cheese and save dozens of calories).
- Choose ham or turkey bacon over bacon and sausage.
- Skip the biscuits, scones, and coffee cake. If you want bread, opt for an English muffin or whole wheat toast.
- Omit the fruit juice, or share a glass if you can't resist fresh squeezed.
- Avoid cream sauces and sugary toppings (syrups), which contribute hundreds of calories to any meal.

Indian

- Tandoori dishes are a good low-fat choice, with lots of spices.
- Choose multiple vegetable (curry) and lentil dishes.
- Avoid fried dishes and coconut sauces.
- Limit the *nan*; once you start it may be hard to stop.

As you can see, beginning the Busy Person's Diet does not have to mean the end of dining out. That would simply not be practical for a busy person! Instead, if you focus on making smart dining-out choices the majority of the time, you can lose weight and still live your life. Now that we have discussed a comprehensive eating strategy, let's move on to the second component of successful weight loss: exercise. Now, don't be tempted to stop reading, insisting that you have no time to exercise. Read on for strategies that even the busiest person can fit into his or her schedule!

FOUR

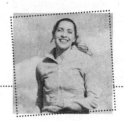

The Busy Person's Exercise Strategies

Grandma didn't exercise. Why must I?

I probably don't need to convince you that getting regular exercise is important for weight loss and even more important for maintenance. But just in case you have any doubts or wonder why your grandmother wasn't an aerobics queen but managed to stay slim, look at how things have changed in the last seventy-five years in this country and throughout the world.

Advances in technology and industrialization may have allowed us to prosper financially, but they have taken a toll on our waistlines. One fascinating study examined the impact of automation on our daily calorie expenditure. The researchers looked at the calories saved daily through the use of common devices like dishwashers, washing machines, escalators, and cars. They found that the average person burned 111 fewer calories per day with these four technological improvements.¹ These advances alone could lead to a five-pound-per-year weight gain if calorie intake is not reduced by an equal amount. Add to that the effect of TV watching and computers, and it is not hard to figure out why we are facing an obesity crisis in this country and all over the world.

I'm not suggesting that you give up your laptop or go back to hand washing your clothes, but to maintain or lose weight, you must make a day-to-day effort to burn more calories to make up for the loss of physical activity due to advances in technology. And since you are reading this book, you probably don't have a lot of time to exercise. So all of my exercise suggestions will be as time efficient as possible.

Getting Your Heart Pumping

Cardiovascular exercise burns the most calories per hour. The number of calories *you* burn depends on your weight, age, fitness level, and exercise intensity. The more you weigh, the more calories you burn doing any activity. Because men usually weigh more than women, they lose more weight through exercise. Older people tend to burn fewer calories than younger, doing the same amount of work. As you age, the pounds don't drop quite as quickly with your regular exercise routine. Finally, people who are more fit burn fewer calories doing the same amount of exercise, but they do burn fat more efficiently.

CALORIES BURNED PER HOUR
FOR THREE DIFFERENT-SIZED PEOPLE
(150-, 200-, and 250-pound persons)

	150	200	250
Aerobics, low impact	345	460	575
Aerobics, step (4 inch)	435	580	725
Aerobics, high impact	510	680	850
Basketball, game	660	880	1,100
Bicycling, 10 mph, light effort	405	540	675
Bicycling, 13 mph, moderate effort	570	760	950
Bicycling, 16 mph, vigorous effort	750	1,000	1,250
Bicycling, stationary, light effort	375	500	625
Bicycling, stationary, moderate effort	480	640	800
Circuit training, general	450	600	750
Golf, general (no cart)	300	400	500
Hiking, cross-crountry	465	620	775
Jumping rope	615	820	1,025
Racquetball, squash	615	820	1,025
Rowing machine	540	720	900
Running, 5 mph (12 min. mile)	555	740	925
Running, 6 mph (10 min. mile)	690	920	1,150
Running, 7 mph (9 min. mile)	825	1,100	1,375
Skating	360	480	600
Skiing, snow, downhill	375	500	625
Skiing, cross-country	660	880	1,100
Stair climbing	420	560	700
Swimming laps, light/moderate effort	360	480	600
Swimming, vigorous (50 yds./min.)	675	900	1,125
Tennis, doubles	315	420	525
Tennis, singles	450	600	750
Walking, 2 mph, slow pace (dog)	180	240	300
Walking, 3 mph, moderate pace	240	320	400
Walking, 4 mph, very brisk pace	300	400	500
Weightlifting, light or moderate effort	210	280	350

Most health experts recommend at least thirty minutes per day of cardiovascular exercise. Recent guidelines suggest that some people may need up to ninety minutes per day of exercise for weight loss and sixty minutes per day for maintenance. Although I don't necessarily disagree, this amount of exercise is impractical for most people, particularly for those with busy lifestyles. I encourage my patients to aim for at least thirty minutes every day or most days of the week. These thirty minutes can be done all at one time or can be divided into three bouts of ten minutes or two bouts of fifteen minutes. Research shows that breaking exercise down into smaller increments does not diminish the benefits and is easier for most people to stick with.[2] If you cannot find the time every day, at least make an effort to exercise more when you do have the time.

Regarding intensity, you should experience some increase in your heart and breathing rates, and conversation should not be easy. Save the bird-watching and window-shopping for your lifestyle exercise (more on that later). If you are always short on time, focus on higher-calorie-burning activities for greatest exercise efficiency. The chart on the previous page shows the approximate calories burned per hour for three different-sized people.

A busy person needs to have a variety of easy cardio options that can consistently fit into his or her day. Ideally, exercise sessions should be scheduled, just like any other appointment. If you can afford it, I highly recommend investing in some type of home exercise equipment. A treadmill, stationary bike, or elliptical machine placed in front of the TV makes it easy to get a half hour of cardio while watching your favorite thirty-minute news show or sitcom. If you are on a budget, a jump rope, workout video, TV exercise program (check out FitTV for lots of options), minitrampoline, or even jumping jacks will work just as well. The key is consistency, and the more easy options a busy person has, the more likely he or she will stick with long-term exercise. For maximum workout efficiency, incorporate interval training into your workouts.

TAKING IT TO THE NEXT LEVEL—INTERVAL TRAINING

Interval training is a great way to keep your workouts interesting, burn more calories in the same amount of time (up to twice the number), and improve your fitness level. Intense intervals should not be done more than two or three times per week, to allow for adequate recovery time. Feel free to modify the interval duration or length of your workouts. Workouts can be done on a treadmill, bike, elliptical machine, or outside. You can build natural intervals into your outdoor workouts by walking, jogging, or biking up and down hills. Be sure to warm up slowly if you are just starting to exercise.

Use the following scale to measure your intensity level:

| Level 1 | Warm-up; gets the blood flowing; breathing is regular |
| Level 2 | Mild pace; breathing and heart rate are slightly increased |

Level 3	Moderate pace; breathing slightly heavier, heart rate rising
Level 4	Challenging pace; breathing hard, conversation difficult, heart rate up
Level 5	Maximum pace; breathing very hard, conversation impossible, heart racing

Basic Interval Workout
  (total workout time = 26–30 minutes)
  1. 3–5-minute warm-up at level 1
  2. 1 minute at level 4
  3. 1 minute at level 2 or 3 (if you are fitter, use level 3)
  4. Repeat steps 2 and 3 for a total of ten intervals = 20 minutes
  5. 3–5-minute cooldown at level 1 or 2

Super Interval Challenge
(total workout time = 18–28 minutes)
  1. 3–5-minute warm-up at level 1
  2. 30-second–1-minute sprint at level 5 (if you are fitter, go for 1 minute)
  3. 1 ½–2 minutes at level 2 or 3—recovery, not rest!
  4. Repeat steps 2 and 3 six times = 12–18 minutes
  5. 3–5-minute cooldown at level 1 or 2

Pyramid Interval Challenge
(total workout time = 20–31 minutes)
  1. 3–5-minute warm-up at level 1

2. 1 minute at level 2
3. 1 minute at level 3
4. 1 minute at level 4
5. 1 minute at level 5
6. 1 minute at level 4
7. 1 minute at level 3
8. 1 minute at level 2
9. Repeat steps 2–8 two or three times = 14–21 minutes
10. 3–5-minute cooldown at level 1

STRENGTH TRAINING AND BEYOND

As discussed earlier, gaining and/or maintaining muscle mass is vital for both weight loss and maintenance. If you don't use your muscles through resistance training while dieting, you are more likely to lose muscle mass, which will decrease your metabolism and make it easier to gain weight back quickly. As you age, it becomes harder to regain lost muscle, so it is best to prevent muscle loss in the first place. If you have never done any strength training, it is never too late to start. Research shows that people can build muscle well into their seventies and eighties.[3]

Resistance training, when done correctly, does not require a major time commitment, which is great for dieters with busy lives. If you go to the gym regularly, I recommend doing a full-body workout (twenty to thirty minutes) two to three times per week. Try to perform one or two exercises per major body part, including back, chest, triceps (back of upper arms), biceps (front of upper arms), shoulders, legs, and abdominals.

Aim for three sets of ten to fifteen per exercise, and use a weight that is challenging but not torturous. If you have never lifted weights before, consider hiring a trainer for a few sessions, to show you proper form. For an even more efficient workout, try not to rest for more than thirty seconds between sets or exercises (also known as circuit training), and you will burn even more calories.

"But I Hate Going to the Gym!"

If you hate the gym or simply don't have the time to get there on a regular basis, a fifteen- to twenty-minute workout can easily be done at home with a set of hand weights, exercise bands, an exercise ball, or even your own body weight. Inexpensive exercise equipment can be purchased at your local sporting goods store or at major discount chains. Many come with instructions on basic exercises, or you can pick up a fitness magazine or book for ideas. One of the best book series for exercise novices is the *Strong Women* series by Dr. Miriam Nelson. If you frequent garage sales, keep your eyes open for exercise books *and* equipment. Well-intentioned people sell their used (or never-used!) exercise machines by the dozens at yard sales. If you are an Internet junkie, community Web sites such as craigslist are also a great place to find used exercise equipment. You may also consider a strength-training workout video or DVD.

If you don't have time for a full-body workout, spend five to ten minutes in the morning or evening and rotate through one or two exercises per day. Or try my favorite technique: perform one exercise during each commercial break, and do as many repetitions or sets as possible in that two-minute period. As you get more advanced or if you are really short on time, find exercises that work two or more body parts simultaneously for the ultimate time-efficient workout!

Beyond Basic Exercise—Yoga, Pilates, and More
Though they require a bit more time, Pilates and more vigorous forms of yoga, such as Bikram and Ashtanga, can also help build and maintain muscle mass. Pilates is especially good for giving muscles a longer, leaner appearance and building core abdominal strength to prevent back injury. Yoga may be particularly beneficial for stress management and stretching to prevent injury and improve balance. You may want to attend a few classes at your local gym or YMCA to learn proper form initially. If time does not allow several classes a week, lots of excellent DVDs are available. For the best selection, go to www.collagevideo.com. My favorite time-efficient DVD series is the Crunch Pilates series, which offers ten minutes per body part (chest, butt, and abs) and the Winsor Pilates twenty-minute workout. The 10 Minute Solution series fits nicely into any schedule.

Burn More All Day
As I explained earlier, lifestyle changes over the past fifty years or so have led to a significant drop in the daily number of calories we burn. To counteract this, we must endeavor as much as possible to increase the number of calories burned through *lifestyle activities*. Lifestyle activities do not burn as many calories per hour as more intentional forms of exercise, like cardio or strength training, but they can add up over the course of a day. Following are examples of lifestyle

activities and the number of calories burned while doing them.

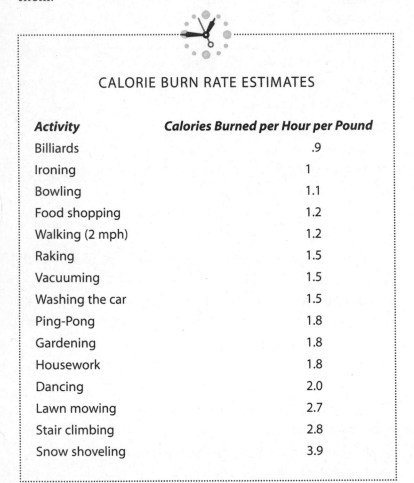

CALORIE BURN RATE ESTIMATES

Activity	Calories Burned per Hour per Pound
Billiards	.9
Ironing	1
Bowling	1.1
Food shopping	1.2
Walking (2 mph)	1.2
Raking	1.5
Vacuuming	1.5
Washing the car	1.5
Ping-Pong	1.8
Gardening	1.8
Housework	1.8
Dancing	2.0
Lawn mowing	2.7
Stair climbing	2.8
Snow shoveling	3.9

THE BUSY PERSON'S LIFESTYLE CHANGES

■ Instead of meeting a friend for drinks, meet for a game of pool or darts (and a drink, if you like).

- Switch to family bowling night instead of family movie night, or go for miniature golf instead of a matinee.
- Always take the stairs.
- Wash your car by hand instead of using the car wash.
- Leave the portable phone on its base instead of by your side on the couch—that way you have to walk to the kitchen to answer it.
- Stand while talking on the phone, instead of sitting.
- Garden, clean, and vacuum whenever you have a chance.
- Volunteer to walk a dog at your local shelter—or get a dog for built-in daily walks.
- Get off the bus or subway two stops earlier, and walk the rest of the way.
- Don't spend five minutes circling the mall or grocery store for the closest parking space. Park in the farthest instead, and burn calories.
- If you are only getting a few things at the market, use a basket instead of a cart.

STAYING MOTIVATED AND PREVENTING BOREDOM

People usually begin exercise programs with great enthusiasm but then often find their motivation quickly dropping off either due to boredom, being busy, or lack of results. Here are a few tips to keep you motivated and prevent workout boredom.

Set Goals. Write down exercise goals, just as you did earlier with weight goals. Make sure your goals are within reach, and gradually set the goals higher to challenge yourself.

(Examples: I will walk 4 times this week; I will go to the gym 3 times; I will run a 5K race within 6 months; I will experiment with a different type of exercise each month.)

Figure out the hows and whens. For the busy person, this is absolutely critical to your success. Each day you should ask yourself *when* and *how*, not *if*, you are going to exercise! If there are obstacles to exercise, work on solutions. If you are traveling, book a hotel with a gym or ask the concierge about local walking routes. If you have evening plans, wake up thirty minutes earlier to squeeze in a quick workout, or go for a walk at lunch.

Track your progress. Keeping track of your workouts (exercises performed and time/repetitions) will reinforce your accomplishments and help you identify areas where you can improve. This does not have to be any more complicated than jotting down items in your food journal.

Buddy up. Find a reliable workout partner. You will be less likely to skip a session when working out with a friend. If you are both competitive, push each other to work harder. It may help to find someone who is already working out regularly to inspire or mentor you.

Match workouts to your personality and lifestyle. Do you live in a cold climate? Then have plenty of indoor workout options, or experiment with fun outdoor options, like snowshoeing or cross-country skiing. Are you the social type? Opt for a team sport, group class at the gym, or golf or tennis game. More of a loner? Build a home gym or go for hikes or bike rides. Have a family? Incorporate them into your exercise routine—dance around the living room with your husband or kids, plan weekend hikes or bike rides, or learn a new sport with the whole family.

Aim for variety, and have fun. Try a new machine or class at the gym. Take tennis or golf instruction. Sign up for salsa lessons. Listen to a new CD or playlist every few weeks. Develop multiple walking routes of different lengths and intensity instead of the same one every day. Not only will this prevent boredom, but you will also be working different muscle groups and thus continuing to improve strength and fitness levels.

Invest in exercise. Treat yourself to a new pair of exercise shoes, a membership to a nice (and convenient) gym, home exercise equipment, a few sessions with a personal trainer, or a high-end pedometer (step counter). Either the financial commitment of regular gym payments/training sessions or the constant workout reminder with those fancy new shoes or pedometer may be just what you need to get or stay motivated!

THE REALITY OF EATING AND EXERCISE

Most of my patients exercise regularly, but very few know how to fuel their bodies correctly to obtain the best possible results. One patient was actually gaining weight while working out up to several hours per day, because she did not understand eating and exercise.

● ● ●

NM was fifty-one years old and perimenopausal when she came to see me three years ago. She was a marathon runner who had stopped training nine months earlier due to an injury and had slowly gained ten pounds. She had just restarted her marathon training and wanted to drop the ten pounds she had gained, but the weight was not coming off despite running up to five times per week. When I checked her metabolism, it was 28 percent below expected based on her age, height, sex, and weight. Her thyroid function was normal, and while I was sure that she had lost some muscle mass after her injury, her metabolism was still surprisingly low. After reviewing her diet, I understood why. As with many other women, NM was drastically undereating while exercising six days a week for at least an hour. Undereating alone can lower metabolism, and undereating *plus* rigorous exercise can throw the body into starvation mode, severely lowering metabolism and causing the body to aggressively hold on to excess body weight.

Much to her surprise, I pushed her to eat more, especially before and after exercise. I kept her starches somewhat low since she was perimenopausal and, therefore, more sensitive to carbohydrates, but I almost doubled the amount of protein she was eating. Within three weeks, she lost five pounds and was beginning to feel better. She found herself waking up hungry, a good sign that her metabolism was recovering. As her workouts increased in length, I encouraged her to increase her starches but to stay away from processed carbohydrates and stick with whole grains, sweet potatoes, and beans. I also encouraged her to add more strength training to regain the muscle she had probably lost after her injury.

Four months later, down seven pounds of fat, I rechecked her metabolism, and this time it was only 2 percent below expected, despite losing weight! As her training sessions became longer and longer, her eating got a bit "sloppy" and she was less organized about meals but tried to adhere to the basic principles 75 percent of the time. Her weight stayed the same.

A year later, because of a back injury, her weight was up a bit. She had tried to watch her food intake carefully and was lifting weights three times a week but had been unable to do much cardiovascular exercise. I checked her body fat percent and found that her muscle mass had actually increased significantly. More important, when I rechecked her metabolism, it was now 26 percent above expected. After analyzing her food journal, her eating was actually more off track than she realized, which was probably why— in spite of her increased metabolism—she had gained a bit of weight. I "tuned up" her diet, and she slowly began dropping weight again, hopefully this time for good!

● ● ●

Carbohydrates are the quickest source of fuel for your body during exercise, and quality protein is important for building muscle and tissue repair. It is important to eat correctly if you really want to optimize your workout, especially if you are exercising strenuously or would like to build more muscle mass. If you plan to exercise intensely or for longer than thirty minutes, and it has been several hours since your last meal, you should try to eat a carbohydrate-containing snack about thirty to forty-five minutes before your workout to keep your energy level up and fuel your workout. Fruit is a terrific option with or without protein. If building muscle is a priority, make sure you eat high-quality protein after your workout. Protein smoothies (homemade or premade) are a great option. They are digested and absorbed quickly, so your body can use them right away.

Unless you are exercising vigorously for more than an hour, you do not need extra calories. While it is important to fuel your body correctly, try not to view exercise as an excuse to eat more.

But here's one caveat: don't eat too many calories just because you're working out. I am always amazed to see people consuming a 250-calorie energy drink or bar after burning 200 calories on the treadmill for twenty or thirty minutes. Don't they realize that, if their goal is weight loss, they just cancelled the calorie-burning benefit of their workout (and more)? If you are trying to lose weight, make sure your pre- and postexercise meals are part of your reduced-calorie regimen, not in addition to regular meals and snacks. Unless you are exercising vigorously for more than an hour, you do not need extra calories. While it is important to fuel your body correctly, try not to view exercise as an excuse to eat more.

I hope this chapter has inspired you to find time to incorporate some type of exercise strategy into your lifestyle. This is without a doubt one of the most critical components of successful, long-term weight loss. Please don't have an all-or-nothing mentality with regard to exercise. Every little thing that you are able to do will add up over time. I know you are busy, but I have yet to meet a patient who could not squeeze in a ten-minute walk here and there—and a couple of sit-ups or push-ups too. If you really think you don't have the time, keep a twenty-four-hour log of your schedule and send it to me. I'll find the time for you!

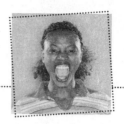

FIVE

The Busy Person's Behavior Tips

I am a weight-loss doctor, not a psychologist. Yet on a daily basis, I deal with eating behavior and psychology with *every one* of my patients. I can't tell you how many new patients come to my office telling me, "I know what to do; I just can't seem to stick with it." For a weight-loss program to be successful for the long-term, particularly for a chronic dieter, diet and exercise are not enough. Behavioral changes are the key to long-term success. Some of these changes may be easy; some may require more work. Based upon my clinical experience, the more changes dieters incorporate permanently, the higher their chances of successful weight loss *and* maintenance.

In this chapter, we will learn some ideas and strategies that have helped many of my patients lose weight successfully. Not every suggestion will apply to you, and you certainly do not have to follow each one precisely to be successful. Focus on those that apply to you the most, and remember that every positive behavior change that you adopt will increase your chances of success.

KEEP A FOOD AND EXERCISE JOURNAL

I refuse to see patients who won't take the time to keep a food and exercise journal. Why? Because writing things down, even just scribbling on a notepad, is a *critical* component of successful weight loss. It is important to write down not only when and what you eat, but also when you exercise. This can help you identify eating issues that you may not have been aware of.

Do you always get hungry two hours after breakfast? Maybe you need more fiber or protein in the morning. Are you famished every day by 4 PM and find yourself grazing until you go to bed? Consider having a larger snack or minimeal around 4 PM to get ahead of your hunger. Have your afternoon workouts been exhausting lately? Maybe you are not taking in enough carbohydrates to fuel your workout. Try adding a piece of fruit forty-five minutes before exercise. By reviewing your journal, you might notice that some food combinations fill you up for longer periods or keep you mentally sharper.

Since people's response to foods is highly variable and I can't review your food journal with you, it's up to you to take my recommendations and optimize them for your body and lifestyle. Each week, try to list in your journal a few observations or things that you would like to work on. More importantly, list a few things that you did well over the past week. When your motivation is low or weight loss slows, look back at your weekly accomplishments and you will probably be pleasantly surprised and proud of how many changes you have made.

Feel free to photocopy the sample food journal page in the back of the book (Appendix E) to use as your weekly journal or go to my Web site (www.drmelina.com) for the food journal that I use in my office. Or just get a small wire-bound notebook and jot down your nutrition and exercise information on a daily basis. Write down any observations and your specific goals on a weekly or biweekly basis.

PRACTICE CHANGING YOUR THINKING

Learn to take things one week at a time, and view your new eating and exercise plan as a journey, not a race, toward a healthier lifestyle. Stop thinking about healthy food as taste-less, exercise as torture, and diet as deprivation. Quit obsess-ing about what you can't eat. Instead, focus on the foods you can and should eat to keep your body running at its peak. It is also important to *believe* that you are capable of change. Have faith in your ability to succeed at weight loss. Try to stay pos-itive, and avoid self-deprecating thoughts—if you constantly tell yourself that you are a failure and will never lose weight, you probably won't. Stay focused on all of the benefits of improving your eating and exercise habits rather than the negatives of failing at another diet. Don't blame genetics, previous diet disappointments, or an unsupportive spouse for your past failure. Concentrate instead on taking control of the future. Remember, your diet and exercise regimen is one of the few things that you can actually *control* in your life, so do it! Stop anguishing over how quickly and seemingly effortlessly your colleagues, friends, spouses, or siblings lost weight. Everyone is different. There are probably things in life that have been easier for you.

Finally, draw on your successes in other aspects of your life to increase your confidence in your ability to lose weight. How did you inspire and motivate yourself to achieve at work? In school? In a personal relationship? Apply successful strategies from these other areas. After all, they worked for you in the past, right? Why not apply them to obtaining a healthy future too?

> Don't blame genetics, previous diet disappointments, or an unsupportive spouse for your past failure. Concentrate instead on taking control of the future. Remember, your diet and exercise regimen is one of the few things that you can actually control in your life, so do it!

DEFINING MISTAKES AND OVERCOMING OBSTACLES

It always surprises me how little my patients think about their mistakes and diet/exercise obstacles until they are in my office. They often come in expecting to lose weight, confidently stating that they had a good eating week. But when the scale hasn't moved much and we review their food journals, they are often astonished at how much more they ate or how little they actually exercised. One patient was shocked to see in her journal that she had had wine or a cocktail with dinner twice as many evenings (and even two lunches) as the previous week, when she had lost a pound. Those extra cocktails probably added up to half a pound that she could have lost. As we discuss the week, patients bring up issues such as these as if it were the first time they even thought about them (it often is). When I ask them to suggest possible solutions, they often come up with several reasonable options on their own. Throughout this book, I have tried to address many of the mistakes and obstacles that my patients bring up regularly. I have also endeavored to present many strategies and solutions.

One of the most common obstacles seems to be a lack of time, which is why it is one of the main foci in this book. But there are many others, so it is essential that you try to analyze what is really getting in the way of your successful weight loss.

■ Do you eat too quickly? Try eating foods that take longer to eat, like soups and salads before each meal.
■ Is your weight-loss strategy too complicated? Simplify your eating as much as possible. Get precut veggies, premade dips and sauces, single-size servings of cheese and nuts, or anything else that will make your diet plan easier.

- Do you overeat in front of the TV at night? Force yourself to only eat in the kitchen or at the dining-room table.
- Does denying your cravings often lead to overeating? Stop trying to "eat around" or satisfy cravings by eating healthier things. Odds are, you will probably end up eating three times as much as you would have if you had just given in to a small serving of what you were really craving.

You are the only one who can define your mistakes and reasons for failure. Work on finding solutions and/or compromises that you can live with over the long-term.

CHEAT SMART

No one can eat perfectly forever. But how you "cheat" matters. Consider a recent patient who had been slowly and steadily losing weight. Her birthday was coming up, and she was very nervous about all the eating-related celebrations to come. When she asked me if it was OK to eat a piece of birthday cake, I told her that I would be more concerned if she did *not* have a piece. She seemed relieved and came in the next week with her biggest weight loss to date. Knowing that she could indulge wisely on occasion had renewed her enthusiasm and commitment to losing weight, and she actually found that she was eating less overall because she was not afraid of feeling deprived.

While nothing should ever be totally off-limits when you are trying to lose weight, most people view eating less-healthy foods as "cheating." I don't particularly like that term, but if you do decide to indulge a bit, it is important to do so correctly so you don't veer off track permanently. First, just deciding to eat something less healthy rather than eating mindlessly is a good start. Don't feel guilty afterward. Guilt leads to negative feelings, which can set in motion negative behavior, such as eating even more unhealthy food.

It is also a good idea to "cheat" publicly. Doing so makes it more acceptable behavior rather than something that you are ashamed of. And finally, try to get right back on track. Don't let one unhealthy meal evolve into an unhealthy day, which turns into an unhealthy week! You probably won't do much damage to your weight-loss efforts with one unhealthy meal, but an entire day can set you back. An entire week can throw you off track permanently.

DON'T WEIGH YOURSELF
MORE THAN ONCE A WEEK

I strongly recommend that you weigh yourself no more than once a week (preferably on the same day, at the same time) for the first few months and every other week thereafter. No matter how perfect your eating and exercise habits are, your weight loss will probably slow a few months into your diet. If you continue to weigh frequently, you may get discouraged or drive yourself crazy chasing a number on the scale. I can't tell you how many times patients come to my office, severely depressed and frustrated after weighing themselves at home *every day*. More often than not, they have lost weight or body fat when I see them, but they spent most of the previous week agonizing over why they were *not* losing weight or second-guessing themselves (and me) because of the daily fluctuations on the scale.

Your scale weight can fluctuate daily due to many different things unrelated to fat loss, including salt intake, hormones, medications, air travel, even weather. It is almost impossible to gain a pound of fat in one day (unless you eat a large pizza and a cheesecake). If your scale goes up a pound in one day, you will probably get agitated or disheartened, which may lead to overeating or, worse, giving up entirely. My most successful patients often get to the point at which they don't even care about the number on the scale. They focus entirely on how their clothes fit, their improvement in energy or health, or how they look in the mirror. They understand that by adopting a healthier lifestyle and making more good daily choices, the scale will usually follow. By weighing yourself weekly or biweekly, you will shift your focus more toward the "big picture" of weight loss and greatly increase your chances of success.

> Your scale weight can fluctuate daily due to many different things unrelated to fat loss, including salt intake, hormones, medications, air travel, even weather.

BUILD AN OPTIMAL WEIGHT-LOSS ENVIRONMENT

It can be useful day by day to optimize both what you can and can't see. Surround yourself with things that remind you of your weight-loss goals, like a photo of you at a healthier weight or your favorite jeans that haven't fit in years, and keep temptation out of sight. One of my patients carries the computer report of her body-fat percentage in her wallet. When she feels her resolve slipping at business lunches, she sneaks a glance at that report. She swears that this helps her always order the healthier choice, no matter how tempting the fried calamari is.

Research shows that when food is visible and accessible, people are more likely to eat more without even realizing it.[1] If your kids must have M&Ms, keep them in a special cabinet that you rarely visit. When a pizza commercial comes on TV, change the channel or browse through a magazine (or better yet, do a few sit-ups). Eat on smaller plates, and drink from tall, narrow glasses to make portions look larger. Visual cues can play an important role in successful weight loss.

MENTALLY REHEARSE CHALLENGING EATING SITUATIONS

Just as professional athletes are often told by their coaches to visualize their performances, you may want to try visualizing your "performance" prior to your next challenging eating situation. If you plan to attend the office happy hour next week at your favorite Mexican restaurant, picture yourself standing far away from the basket of chips and giant bowl of guacamole and enjoying the conversation rather than mindlessly gorging, as you have in the past. You still seem to be having fun, don't you? Now, as a result of your self-control here, picture yourself looking great at the beach or gym next summer, instead of wearing the baggy shirt and shorts again!

Maybe you have been dreading your best friend's wedding next month; your date just cancelled, and you know *someone* will ask when *you* are getting married. Add to that the open bar and plentiful hors d'oeuvres, and it could easily spell trouble. So, picture yourself opting for mineral water with lime, and just a glass or two of champagne instead of the five tequila shots you planned on. Now see yourself spending the evening twirling around the dance floor, even if it is with the bride's five-year-old niece. Isn't it nice to wake up the next morning feeling energetic and lean?

Mentally rehearsing how you handle challenging situations can help make your success a reality. And painting a visual picture of the consequences of your choices, both negative and positive, can also be useful. You may even want to develop a special motivational phrase or image to help you when you find yourself in different eating situations. There is a reason these strategies work for athletes. Why not incorporate them into your weight-loss effort too?

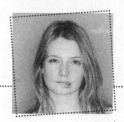

SIX

The Busy Person's Real-World Challenges

I had a patient recently who was doing terrific following the Busy Person's Diet. He had lost twenty-five pounds, felt great, and had even dropped his cholesterol 20 points. Then he went on vacation to Mexico. He figured that a few margaritas a day, breakfast pastries each morning, and cheese-laden dinners couldn't be too terrible, right? He deserved a break from exercise and spent leisurely days lying on the beach, with an occasional dip in the pool. He rationalized that he was on vacation, so he was going to relax and truly enjoy himself.

Ten days later, he came back five pounds heavier. Shocked and a bit depressed, he vowed that on future vacations he would allow for some indulgence, but never again would he "turn off" everything he had learned through the

Busy Person's Diet. It just did not seem worth it anymore after years of struggling to lose.

Taking The Busy Person's Diet on the Road

Vacation and travel are two of the most challenging circumstances for people trying to lose weight. The lack of routine and structure can easily derail even the most dedicated nutrition and exercise plan. Whether you are traveling for business or pleasure, it is important to plan ahead and try to adopt some of the following strategies.

For most people, vacations and business travel usually lead to weight gain, unless perhaps you are trekking in Nepal. Be realistic about weight and travel expectations. Most people do expect to gain while traveling. But while it is unlikely that you will lose weight on vacation, maintaining your weight is not at all unreasonable.

> For most people, vacations and business travel usually lead to weight gain, unless perhaps you are trekking in Nepal. Be realistic about weight and travel expectations.

I strongly discourage cutting calories drastically to lose extra weight prior to vacations. This may slow metabolism and lead to more rapid weight gain when you start eating normally during your trip. You will also probably be starving and feeling deprived; you may be even more likely to overeat during your trip. Don't set yourself up for failure before you even head to the airport. Speaking of air travel, here are a few travel tips.

- Don't take the airport's moving walkway or escalator. It always amazes me to see people sitting quietly in the waiting area for hours prior to departure, or taking the conveyor when they have a roller bag. Remember, you will be sitting for hours. Why not burn a few extra calories and walk wherever you can? Window-shop while you wait, or just walk laps around the terminal. Or maybe do some discreet knee bends or calf raises in the waiting area. Anything to make up for the calories you *won't* burn stuck on a plane for hours.
- Bring healthy snacks for the flight, like nuts, protein bars, or fruit. Or eat a satisfying meal, like a sandwich or salad, at the airport instead of loading up on snack food during the plane trip.
- Drink water. Hunger and thirst can feel similar, and air travel can dehydrate you, so drink plenty of water and minimize alcohol and caffeine consumption on travel days. These can also dehydrate you.

Now that you have arrived at your destination, whether you are on business or taking that vacation you planned for months, try the following suggestions. Sticking to even a few could mean the difference between fitting into your pants on the trip home or not!

- Don't deprive yourself. If you're on vacation, live a little. Just try to make choices on what you will splurge on. If you feel like dessert or wine, skip the bread and potatoes. If you are craving bread, limit yourself to one or two pieces, and skip dessert. Try to splurge on unique, regional food items and house specialties, not chips or junk food.

- Avoid sugary beverages and cocktails. Skip the daily fresh juice, lemonade, or soda. If you drink alcohol, stick with wine, beer, or spirits with club soda, diet soda, or lime. A big glass of orange juice could easily cancel out the calories you burned during that lovely morning walk. Margaritas and daiquiris contain up to 500 calories and can easily pack on one to two pounds a week. Is it really worth it? Treat yourself to one on your first day; then make the choice not to drink your calories for the rest of the trip.

- Find ways to get extra physical activity each day. Swim, snorkel, bike the countryside, go for walks after dinner, go dancing, or shop. You don't have to frequent the hotel gym in Hawaii or Paris, but make a conscious effort to do more lifestyle-based activity. Or consider taking an active or fitness vacation if you are feeling especially motivated or adventurous. Many of my patients have gone on hiking trips to keep up their healthy habits or spent a week at a tennis camp instead of lying on the beach. If you are traveling on business, consider staying at a hotel that has in-room fitness options or a gym. Many hotels now cater to fitness-minded business travelers. Or pack an exercise band and jump rope in your suitcase and do a few exercises and stretches at night.

■ Don't forget the basics. Even while on vacation or traveling, try to stick with protein-based meals and snacks, high-quality carbohydrates, reasonable portions, and regular exercise. Also, do your best to plan ahead and make sure you have access to what you need. If your hotel has a fridge, find a local market and get some cottage cheese and fruit to snack on. Or bring nuts and fruit to the pool or sightseeing. One of my patients ships a box of healthy food ahead every time she visits her mother in South America, to make sure she always has healthy choices to balance out the heavier food her family often cooks.

■ When you get home, go food shopping as soon as possible. Since you probably did not lose weight on vacation, it is important to get right back on track with your nutrition program. By filling the house with healthy food right away, you will have no excuse. Here's how one of my patients, a frequent traveler, managed to lose more than fifty pounds despite regular trips to tropical locations!

● ● ●

GM is a perky sixty-year-old woman who came to see me at the suggestion of her doctor. Other than having slightly high cholesterol and blood pressure, she was quite healthy but was carrying an extra sixty to seventy pounds on her petite five-foot-three-inch frame. She had been steadily gaining weight since her late twenties and had had moderate success with Weight Watchers but had slowly regained the weight she had lost and a bit more. The previous year, she had walked an hour a day but stopped because she had not seen any results on the scale. She was definitely a "carb person," and a typical day often included cereal for breakfast, a burrito for lunch, and cereal or a large restaurant meal for dinner. She was taking lots of vitamins, half of which she could not remember why she was taking but thought she must have read something that indicated that they were useful.

Her husband traveled frequently on business, and she occasionally accompanied him. They also often traveled together for pleasure. When her husband was in town or when they were both away, they went out for nice dinners almost every night. When she was home alone, she never cooked for herself. I told her that my approach was perfect for her since it did not require any cooking and allowed for eating out and travel.

Since she fit the criteria for metabolic syndrome, I cut her starches dramatically, starting her out at two to three per day. To prevent hunger, I increased her protein intake moderately. She agreed to eat regularly throughout the day. She also agreed to start walking again. (Note: Research has shown that alone—without a reduced-calorie diet—walking or any other exercise will not lead to weight loss in women.)

After two weeks, she had dropped almost three and a half pounds and felt really good. She was not hungry and did not feel obsessed with food as she had when dieting in the past. I encouraged her to start some form of resistance training to ensure that she did not lose muscle since it is harder to rebuild as you age. After a little more than a month, and down seven pounds, she had to travel to Boston for a long weekend with her husband. She was nervous about getting off track. "This is the best I've ever done," she said. I assured her that if she stuck to the basics and planned ahead, she would be fine. I gave her my travel handout and sent her off.

She came back a week later down another one and a half pounds and thrilled at how well she had eaten during her trip, with a little planning and a few compromises at dinner. She even had her husband exercising with her over the weekend. Three weeks later, she was off to Hawaii for Thanksgiving, and this time she was confident in her ability to stay on track. She was up to five days a week of walking and found that chocolate-flavored premade protein drinks were great between meals. By the time she left for Hawaii, she was down another five and a half pounds, and her confidence was increasing on a weekly basis. She decided to bring protein drinks with her to Hawaii for easy breakfasts or snacks and worked out on the treadmill every day (I would have walked on the beach instead, but everyone has preferences). Despite slightly indulgent but careful nightly restaurant dinners, she returned a few weeks later more than three pounds lighter.

Over the holidays, she went back to Hawaii but stayed on track by eating mainly salads with protein, protein drinks, and fruit and exercising regularly. One month later she was five pounds lighter, much happier, more energetic, and looking terrific. Down more than twenty pounds, she now had the blood pressure of a twenty-year-old. We decided to see each other monthly at this point, since she was feeling so self-assured and on track with her eating. After another month her weight loss slowed a bit to half a pound each week. I assured her that this was normal but gave her my plateau-busters handout to help her troubleshoot. After reading my suggestions, she decided to increase the intensity of her workouts by walking faster and dancing. She also started measuring her nut servings again and realized that she may have been overdoing it a bit. After two weeks of making these changes, she had lost another two and a half pounds, breaking through her slight weight-loss plateau.

Over the next few months, despite frequent travel, she lost another seven pounds, which brought her total loss to fifty pounds. At this point, she hit another plateau and actually went up a few pounds. After reviewing her food journal, I found that she was eating too many nuts again, and I encouraged her to switch to vegetables and hummus or an apple for snacks instead. I also suggested that she spice up her exercise routine and recommended that she try my favorite Pilates DVD by Crunch Fitness. She followed all of my suggestions and got right back on track, losing in less than a month the few pounds that she had gained.

THE BUSY PERSON ON WEEKENDS

My office is located in San Francisco, less than an hour from wine country. Many of my patients work in high-stress jobs during the week and love to relax on weekends in Napa Valley or Sonoma. This relaxation usually involves great wine and great food—and both can wreak havoc on their diets. While I would never discourage patients from enjoying themselves in arguably one of the most beautiful areas in the country, I spend a lot of time helping them figure out ways to minimize the damage that indulgent weekend eating and drinking can do to their diets. A few simple choices can be the difference between slow, steady weight loss and taking two steps forward, two steps back.

I know that weekends can be challenging when you are trying to lose or maintain weight. I hear this story on a regular basis: "I've worked hard all week, exercised regularly, planned my meals and snacks, finished that big project at work, drove the kids to and from all of their activities, and now I feel I *deserve* to loosen up a little over the weekend. How much harm can I really do in two and a half days?"

A *lot*. An extra 250 calories per day (the equivalent of one glass of wine and a small cookie) on Friday, Saturday, and Sunday can add up to a thirteen-pound weight gain per year, or prevent a thirteen-pound weight loss, if consumed on a regular basis. And research shows that the average nineteen- to seventy-year-old eats 115 calories *more* each weekend day (Friday to Sunday), amounting to about a five-pound-per-year weight gain.[1] Interestingly, the same study also found that all of the increased calories come from fat and alcohol, not protein and carbohydrates. Take that into consideration when you are reaching for that second serving of wine and cheese.

What does this mean to you? While there is room for occasional indulgences, helping to prevent feelings of deprivation and cravings, the key is *keeping* them occasional—and moderate. Don't "let go" entirely on weekends. If you do, you will constantly be taking two steps forward and one—or two—steps back. This can slow your progress considerably and be very discouraging over the long-term. I don't expect you to eat exactly the same, seven days a week, but there are a few strategies I recommend to help you avoid some common mistakes and keep some control over the weekends. Many of these will look familiar; they apply to any challenging situation. But they are so important that they are worth repeating.

PLAN, PLAN, PLAN

Weekends tend to be less structured than weekdays at work, so people often don't eat regular meals. Or they find themselves so busy running errands that they don't stop for food for hours. Don't let this happen. Think ahead. It's much harder to take the time to find a healthy meal or snack when you are famished and everything sounds good.

- Try to eat a satisfying breakfast before heading out the door.
- Always carry a protein bar, a small bag of nuts, or a piece of fruit with you.
- At the very least, make sure to consider healthy eating options before you feel famished.
- Plan out your evenings too. If you are going out to dinner or a party, cut back on your starches and fat during the day since you will likely eat more of each when dining away from home. But don't starve yourself all day to gorge at night. You will probably be so hungry by the time dinner comes that you will eat twice as many calories in half the time.

DRINK ALCOHOL WISELY

Since research shows that excess weekend calories often come from alcohol, it makes sense to limit alcohol if you are trying to lose weight.[2] While I have seen no research indicating that alcohol stimulates appetite, it can lower willpower and make healthier choices seem far less appealing. Some of my patients prefer to eliminate alcohol entirely while they are trying to lose weight, but avoiding alcohol completely is not necessary for most. Some patients actually make better choices if they have a cocktail or glass of wine before or with dinner. It seems to relax them and decrease stress- or anxiety-driven eating choices. This does not mean that you should start drinking if you do not drink alcohol. But if you find a glass of wine relaxing, you do not necessarily have to eliminate it for successful weight loss. Whatever strategy works best for you, do not forget that alcohol has almost double the calories per gram of carbohydrates and protein. If you do choose to drink over the weekend, you must cut calories elsewhere to compensate.

EXTEND YOUR EXERCISE

I'm always astounded when patients tell me they did not exercise over the weekend because they "just wanted to relax." Weekends are the best time to exercise, especially for someone with a busy life, because you probably have more time over the weekend than during the week. Motivate yourself to do more activity, not less, over the weekend. Wear a pedometer and see how many steps you can accumulate on weekend days. Challenge yourself to increase your total by a few hundred steps each weekend. Weather permitting, take the family on a long hike or bike ride to make up for the mini bouts of exercise you squeezed in during the hectic week. Sign up for that yoga class you have been considering for months. Or head to the mall and walk around window-shopping for an hour before letting yourself buy something. Instead of eating an extra 115 calories a weekend, like the average adult American, challenge yourself to *burn* an extra 115 calories. You could lose five extra pounds in one year, without doing anything else!

AIM TO MAINTAIN ON WEEKENDS

While I encourage patients not to "let go" on weekends, I understand that weekends are a time to relax a bit and socialize. Many of my patients find it easier to approach weekends with the goal of maintaining their weight rather than being strict in their effort to lose weight. Though consistency is key, finding the balance between consistency and liveability is essential. If you enjoy having dessert or an extra glass of wine on weekends, or perhaps a less restrictive brunch, go ahead. Just make sure that you don't go completely overboard and have six cocktails, a large slice of cheesecake, and French toast loaded with syrup the next day. I don't recommend taking a "day off" or even an entire meal "off" as some diets recommend, but a planned indulgence will not interfere significantly with your weight loss in the short- or long-term and may even help you mentally stay on track.

THE BUSY PERSON DURING THE HOLIDAYS

I love the holidays and usually have lots of free time to enjoy them since most of my patients avoid both me and the scale during the month of December (almost as much as they avoid stale holiday fruitcakes!). Studies show that while the average American gains only a pound or two between Thanksgiving and New Year's, those with weight problems often gain five to ten pounds.[3] But don't despair. Many of my patients have successfully maintained their weight over the holidays and a rare few have even lost weight. I encourage most patients to focus on maintenance during December since it is such a challenging time of year, with so much temptation and so many time demands. As always, the key to success is planning. Here are several strategies to safely get you through this difficult time of year without sustaining too much of a blow to your weight-loss effort:

Never go to a party or dinner starving. Eat a protein-based, high-fiber snack or minimeal beforehand to take the edge off your appetite. Try turkey slices wrapped in a low-carb tortilla, cottage cheese and an apple, a high-fiber protein bar, or nonfat yogurt with one-fourth cup of high-fiber cereal. If you plan to drink alcohol, you may want to include a little fat in your snack, like nuts or string cheese. Fat slows the absorption of alcohol into your bloodstream.

Set the stage for success. Believe it or not, several aspects of your holiday eating "stage" are under your control. Instead of hoping for healthy eating choices, bring your own. A vegetable tray with low-fat dip is always a good idea. And if you want to have a little dessert, why not bring a fruit tray with yogurt and honey dip, or even low-fat minicupcakes (built-in portion control)? Before hitting the buffet line or hors d'oeuvres, survey the entire spread to figure out ahead of time your best options and potential splurges. By doing this, you will optimize your eating choices instead of mindlessly putting things on your plate as you encounter them. Finally, after filling your plate, park yourself away from the food table for the rest of the night. The closer you are, the more tempted you will be to grab a few more miniquiches or cookies. Believe me, proximity to food matters.

Watch alcohol intake closely. Alcohol is not only filled with empty calories (one cup of eggnog, a Christmas favorite, has 300 calories and 22 grams of fat!), but it can also make self-control at the Christmas cookie table virtually impossible. Make sure to drink plenty of water before a dinner or party, and try alternating a glass of water or sparkling water (not juice or soda, which has loads of calories) with each alcoholic beverage. Also, avoid sugary mixers such as juice and soda, as these add hundreds of sugar calories.

Squeeze in time for exercise/activity. The holidays are generally a season when not even the most devoted gym buff has time to exercise. Unfortunately for those with weight issues, the holidays are one of the most important times to increase or, at the very least, maintain exercise to prevent weight gain. Be creative and find as many ways as possible to be more active. Force yourself to use only the stairs when shopping at the mall or department store. Do push-ups, sit-ups, and jumping jacks while watching TV. Go for a walk before or after Christmas or Thanksgiving dinner. Plan active outings with family and friends. If you don't have time to get to the gym, get a jump rope and commit to five minutes daily. Organize a family dance contest after dinner. Volunteer to wash dishes or clean the house before or after your family's holiday dinner. If after-work holiday parties interfere with exercise, take a walk at lunch or before work. Do anything you can to burn more calories.

Use the two-thirds-party-plate strategy. Fill two-thirds of your plate with lean protein and veggies. Use the remaining one-third for the special, delicious, and not-so-good-for-you items. Don't avoid them. You will just feel deprived and overeat later! And don't waste calories on the fillers: rolls, chips, cheese, and crackers that you can eat any time of year.

Make trade-offs. Skip wine at one party, and skip dessert at another. If you have a little pasta or bread, limit yourself to one glass of wine instead of two. Before or after any big dinner or party, cut back on starch and fat, since that is more than likely what you will eat too much of. You can be social and enjoy yourself while remaining in control of your eating. Ask yourself how much stuffing, pie, cakes, cookies, bread, and chocolate you have eaten in past Christmases and Thanksgivings. Do you really need more of everything? Choose just your favorites this year, and skip the rest. If you feel your resolve slipping, focus on how great you are going to feel in January when you have not gained weight for the first time in . . . how many years?

Get rid of leftovers. If you are having a party, make sure to send guests home with the leftover Christmas cookies and treats. Not only will they appreciate the holiday spirit, but you won't be faced with the cookie tray for the next four days. If your family protests, compromise and let them keep one serving of their favorite in a special part of the fridge or cabinet.

Dress the part. Don't wear loose-fitting clothes to a party or dinner. This may sound ridiculous, but if your clothes have plenty of room for expansion, you may not realize how stuffed you are getting, and you will be less aware of your expanding waistline. Any tactic you can use to get through the holidays without gaining ten pounds is worth trying, right?

WHEN THE SCALE WON'T BUDGE

Weight-loss plateaus are an almost inevitable part of weight loss. There is no single reason why they occur in any individual, but there are several possible explanations. Weight loss may temporarily, or permanently, stop due to changes in your body chemistry, muscle mass, or metabolism. Research has shown that dieters who restrict calories too drastically can decrease their metabolism within forty-eight hours.[4] In addition, obese people who have lost more than 10 percent of their body weight often have a greater drop in metabolism than expected. You must also remember that as you lose weight, your body requires fewer calories, so to prevent plateaus, you must eat a little less or exercise a little more to continue losing weight steadily.

From a behavior standpoint, the longer a person follows a restricted eating plan, the more seemingly harmless calories may sneak into their daily eating plan. Just as small changes can add up over time to weight loss, small increases in daily calorie intake can prevent weight loss over time.

Finally, exercise frequency and duration often decreases over time as enthusiasm diminishes.

Plateau Busters

Taking into consideration all the potential causes for weight-loss plateaus, here are some tips to help you break through that frustrating plateau quickly so you are not tempted to abandon your goals entirely. Many of these will also help you lose those last ten pounds if you find yourself struggling.

Go back to the basics. Write down everything you eat for one week. If you have already been recording your food intake, be more vigilant. Try to figure out if an extra 50 to 100 calories (or more) may be sneaking in each day and adding up over a week or two to prevent you from losing weight. When I review the journals of most of my patients who have stopped losing, I find that higher fat and starchy food portions have crept up a bit or the frequency of little splurges has increased slightly. Usually, "cleaning up" a bit is enough to kick their weight loss back into gear.

Cut bread for a week. This strategy has helped many of my patients, especially peri- and postmenopausal women, break through weight-loss plateaus. For some, it may be necessary to restrict bread during the remainder of your weight-loss plan and reintroduce it carefully during maintenance.

Spice it up. Try adding more spices to meals. Spicier foods, like hot peppers, may rev up your metabolism. In addition, more flavorful foods tend to be more satisfying, so you may fill up with less food. Try adding cinnamon, cumin, cardamom, chili powder, fennel, and anything else you can think of to soups, veggies, and sauces. At the very least, your food will taste a lot better!

Double your vegetables. For some reason, no matter how quick, tasty, and easy I try to make eating vegetables, they seem to be the first food group that drops off over time. For this reason, whenever a patient stops losing weight and insists that nothing has changed in his diet, my first piece of advice is to double his intake of nonstarchy vegetables for a week. This strategy often does the trick for busting through a weight-loss plateau.

Add intervals. Interval training workouts, described earlier, are a great way to kick up the intensity of your exercise, no matter what your level of fitness is. As I explained, the more fit you are, the fewer calories you burn doing the same exercise. By adding intervals, you burn more calories in the same amount of time. If you have not tried intervals, now is the time to start. If you are already including interval training in your workout routine, increase the intensity of your intervals by increasing the duration or speed of the intervals or the resistance or incline of the machine.

Change things up. Change your cardio and weight routine every six to eight weeks. You do not have to make drastic changes, but by doing a different type of exercise that uses different muscle groups (or the same muscle groups in a different way), you can often break through or prevent weight-loss plateaus. If you have been walking, try biking, or hop on the elliptical machine for ten minutes. If you have been walking flat trails, add hills; or walk for two minutes, jog for two minutes, and keep alternating.

With resistance training, try learning a new exercise for each body part or increasing your weight or the number of repetitions per set. If you are using bands, increase the tension. If you belong to a gym, treat yourself to a few personal training sessions to learn good technique. And if your weight goes up a bit initially but your clothes feel looser, don't worry; that means that you are building muscle and losing fat, both of which are essential for long-term success.

Don't deprive yourself entirely. If you have been craving an apple fritter for six months, have one (or half of one) and get it out of your system. Plan small indulgences here and there. Often the mental satisfaction can help get you back on track. In trying to avoid that temptation for so long, you may have been eating more than you realized.

Change up your diet. If you have been eating the same thing every day for breakfast and/or lunch, try something different for a week or two. If you have too much variety in your diet, keep things a little simpler for a week or two. You can also try alternating slightly higher-calorie days with lower-calorie days or slightly higher-carbohydrate days with lower-carb days. For example, if you have been eating three starches daily, try to cut down to one or two for a day or two each week. Or cut fat intake in half for a day, and have a bit more in place of carbohydrates the next day. This may help kick-start your weight loss.

Stay positive. This is probably one of the most important suggestions. It is critical that you try not to obsess if your weight loss has temporarily stopped. Don't weigh yourself daily, agonizing over the number on the scale. This will only depress you and likely cause you to crave the foods that will prevent you from losing weight. Trust me, I know that it is difficult when you feel you are doing everything right but the scale is not cooperating. But if you have adhered to these suggestions and are carefully watching what you eat and exercising more, your weight will eventually begin to drop again, especially if you try to stay positive and not let the number on the scale define you.

Here is how one of my patients, who had struggled with weight since the age of ten, lost more than eighty pounds by slowly and steadily working through numerous plateaus.

● ● ●

JP came to see me at the age of forty-one. At five-foot-seven and 332 pounds, he would be a challenge. His traveling food-sales job and part-time chef work did not help. He was on the road five days a week. On weekends he loved to ride his Harley around town with his buddies, who didn't exactly have the greatest eating habits. His typical eating day included no breakfast, fast-food lunch (burger, fries, Coke), and late dinners, which he either prepared or picked up on his way home. He also had frequent "chef's dinners" as a member of the local culinary institute. His exercise involved walking to accounts for up to seven hours, three days a week. He wanted to lose more than a hundred pounds and get to a weight he had not seen since 1979.

JP was pretty healthy and active. His blood sugar and blood

pressure were a little high and his thyroid was a little low, but he had no other significant medical problems. I decided to gradually ease him into a healthier way of eating and told him not to expect overnight changes since he had struggled with weight his entire life. He began eating breakfast regularly, sometimes having a protein shake, sometimes cereal. For lunch, he had a sandwich or salad instead of fast food, and dinners did not change much; he just cut the starchy carbohydrates, like bread, pasta, rice, and potatoes. It was hard finding the time to exercise, so I chose to focus more on his diet initially. He survived the holidays and actually lost five pounds between Thanksgiving and Christmas. I knew we were on the right track.

After six months, JP had lost twenty-five pounds, certainly not rapid weight loss, but at least he was consistent. Over the next six months, he went up and down five to ten pounds several times. He was skipping meals again and was still not exercising, but I didn't give up, and neither did he. At this point, he decided to check out a local gym that was relatively convenient for him on his work route. He tried a kickboxing class and was hooked. He began kickboxing two to three times a week, and the weight started slowly coming off again. Over the next six months, he lost another twenty-five pounds and was starting to notice a big difference in his energy level. His blood sugar was now totally normal, and he had lost seven inches off his waist size.

Over the next six months, JP slowly lost another thirty-two pounds, another seven inches off his waist, and his blood pressure was now normal. He went to the gym at least twice most weeks and ate three meals daily and an afternoon snack most of the time. If his weight increased, rather than get discouraged, we worked together to troubleshoot. At one point he was not eating enough protein, and his weight didn't budge until we added the protein shakes back into his diet. At another plateau, we spent two visits trying to figure out what was going on. I finally got to the bottom of things: he had started drinking Gatorade on the road, thinking that since it was much healthier than soda, it was OK. I explained to him that the sugar content and calories in Gatorade were not much different from soda, and he simply did not need that much sugar. He switched to diet soda and began losing weight again.

Another six months passed, and JP slowly lost another ten pounds and another two inches off his waist. His total weight loss over the two and a half years that I worked with him was eighty-three pounds. At this point, he decided to change jobs and moved out of state. We keep in touch, and he has maintained the weight loss and lifestyle. He did not reach his goal weight, but his patience, dedication, and commitment to a healthier lifestyle were inspiring, and I'm sure he looks a whole lot better riding his Harley around his new town.

BEATING THE BINGEING GAME

Binge eating is fairly common among chronic dieters and overweight and obese people. *Bingeing* is defined as experiencing a lack of control that leads to eating a very large amount of food within a two-hour period. Binges are usually associated with eating very quickly, eating until you are uncomfortably full, eating when you aren't hungry, eating alone because of embarrassment over the amount of food you consume, and feeling ashamed and depressed after a binge.[5] If episodes like this happen to you regularly (twice a week or more), talk with your doctor about seeing a psychologist. If you experience such occurrences less frequently, do your best to prevent these types of situations by applying the following recommendations.

Avoid trigger foods in high-risk situations. Eating just a small amount of tasty food can cause significant cravings, so it is important to avoid those beloved and supertasty foods if you have had a few drinks or are feeling depressed or stressed-out. Obviously, the best way to avoid these foods is to not have them in the house. The effort of having to go out and get something may just be enough to prevent the binge.

If you do binge, force yourself to eat only at the dining room or kitchen table, and avoid eating directly out of containers. By transferring foods to bowls or plates, you maintain some portion control, which can prevent the mindless overeating that bingeing often involves. If you allow yourself to eat while watching TV, you are making it much easier to detach yourself from your eating and much more difficult to stop eating before the major damage is done.

What caused the binge? It may be helpful to write down why you did it and how it made you feel afterward so you can look back at it the next time you feel vulnerable. Also, try to figure out nonfood strategies when you find yourself in similar situations. Maybe you can designate a "binge buddy," a close friend you call when you are tempted. Do anything you can to keep busy: clean, walk the dog, paint your nails, wash your car—anything to derail the bingeing behavior.

Try to visualize how you would look and feel after a bingeing episode, and then visualize how you would look and feel after preventing one and, by doing so, moving one step closer to your weight-loss goals. Again, much like professional athletes mentally rehearse their performance, mentally rehearse avoiding a binge and waking up a winner.

Finally, after a binge, it is essential that you forgive yourself and focus on getting back on track. Do not torture yourself by getting on the scale the next morning or trying on the pants that fit you perfectly two days ago. This will only dispirit you, making you more susceptible to bingeing again.

● ● ●

JS is a great example of the fact that exercise alone does not necessarily lead to weight loss. He is a successful attorney in his late thirties who came to see me for weight loss, despite following a vigorous cycling training and exercise regimen. He had struggled with weight since second grade and had peaked at more than 300 pounds during law school. He is an avid cyclist, and when the weather is good, he usually goes on serious bike rides on the weekends, riding three or more hours on a regular basis. During the week, his bike is set up on a trainer in the living room to get in a few more days of training.

Despite this high level of activity, he was sixty to seventy pounds heavier than he felt he should be for optimal cycling performance and had not found an eating approach that balanced fueling his body for a high-performance level with weight loss. His eating habits were fairly typical for a busy male, and he often ate 75 percent of his daily calories at night. He complained of always feeling hungry and felt that starches often set him off on eating binges.

The first few changes I made to his diet were to increase his protein intake (to decrease his constant hunger) and to make sure he ate both morning and afternoon protein-based snacks so he did not come home famished and polish off the entire plate of fresh-baked cookies that his wife had prepared for their daughters. These changes seemed to help, and he dropped five pounds quickly. He felt very good about not being hungry all the time and found that the afternoon snack was critical.

Next, we focused on eating before and after his long weekend rides, after which he often complained of overwhelming cravings. I emphasized the importance of adequate carbohydrate intake before, during, and after any workout longer than ninety minutes. He had been avoiding eating too many carbs after long rides since his workout was complete, and he did not think he needed the extra fuel. I explained to him the importance of quickly replenishing his muscle glycogen, the storage form of sugar, through adequate carbohydrate intake. In fact, his strong carbohydrate cravings may have been his body's way of signaling him to "refill the fuel tank."

Over the next six weeks, he worked on optimizing his pre- and postworkout meals and in the process lost fourteen pounds. A few weeks later, down another five pounds, he found that he was really craving pizza and obsessing about it. I assured him that it was fine to have pizza in moderation. After all, this was a lifestyle, not a diet. He planned to indulge the next weekend after a long bike ride but came in the following week regretting his decision. He hadn't really wanted the pizza after his ride, but he ate it anyway since he had already planned on it. He didn't feel well for a few days, and he admitted to a minibinge of cookies and chocolate the night before coming in to see me. I encouraged him to do everything he could to turn off his all-or-nothing mentality, assuring him that this was very common among my patients, especially the more successful, goal-oriented, type-A personalities.

He agreed to be a bit less rigid with food choices and got right back on track, losing another six pounds over the next month. At this point, he was in a weight range that he had not seen in years and was feeling great. He was easily riding sixty-five miles a day on weekends, but he decided he wanted to lose weight faster. He cut back on his eating over the next two weeks and, not surprisingly, binged the night before coming in to see me. His weight had not budged. I again emphasized that deprivation usually leads to bingeing. I recommended that he stop focusing on the number on the scale and focus more on his performance and controlling his eating without trying to eat perfectly.

JS went on to lose an additional 7 ½ pounds and realized the cycling goals that had motivated him to lose weight. While he did not reach his goal weight and still struggles with occasional eating challenges, he has maintained a forty-pound weight loss for several years, and I'm confident that he will never allow himself to return to the starting weight he had when he first came to see me.

STAYING ON TRACK

In my weight-loss practice, my patients are often very motivated during the first month or two that they see me, when the weight is coming off steadily, stress levels are relatively manageable, and the eating and exercise plan is new and interesting. But after the first few months, many begin to lose motivation and focus. Whether due to boredom, time constraints, an indulgent weekend, a stressful work deadline, or slower weight loss, getting off track is very common. You may find that you are making more and more poor choices each week. Or maybe you are finding less and less time to exercise or be active. Perhaps you went on vacation and couldn't get back into the swing of things on your return. Or maybe you have become bored with eating the same types of things every day or tired of feeling that you have to watch what you eat all the time. If any of the above applies to you or you simply need a little mental boost, this is a good time to reidentify your motivation, reset your goals, and refocus your efforts. I have developed a worksheet to help you with this task.

POSITIVE CHANGES I HAVE MADE
IN THE PAST FEW MONTHS

Make sure to set aside a little time to fill this out. Don't just scribble down a few responses. Really think about what a healthy lifestyle change and permanent weight loss mean to you. List the positive eating, exercise, and behavioral

changes you have made in the past few months. If you have
been using the weekly worksheets, refer back to these to
refresh your memory. Otherwise, look through your food
journal or just think back on your eating, exercise, and behavior prior to starting this program. Feel free to include even
the smallest accomplishments, like "skipped dessert twice
last week" or "walked up the stairs to use the restroom on the
next floor two weeks ago."

1. _____

2. _____

3. _____

4. _____

5. _____

REAL REASONS I WANT TO LOSE WEIGHT

List old or new reasons why you want to lose weight (refer
back to the reasons you listed in Chapter 2). What does losing

weight, exercising more, and being healthier really mean to you?

1. _____

2. _____

3. _____

4. _____

5. _____

My Short- and Long-Term Goals

Set several realistic and fun short- and long-term goals (run two miles without stopping, get to the gym three times a week for the next month, fit into a size ____ pair of pants by Christmas, learn a new and easy vegetable recipe that you *love*, find a healthy new restaurant near the office, etc.).

1. _____

2. _____

3. _____

4. _____

5. _____

Define a few diet, exercise, and behavior problem areas and try to address one of them each week for the next six weeks.

Week 1 problem area:

_____

How I plan to work on it:

_____

_____

Week 2 problem area:

_____

How I plan to work on it:

_____

_____

Week 3 problem area:

_____

How I plan to work on it:

_____

_____

Week 4 problem area:

_____

How I plan to work on it:

_____

_____

Week 5 problem area:

_____

How I plan to work on it:

_____

_____

Week 6 problem area:

_____

How I plan to work on it:

_____

_____

Hopefully after completing this worksheet, you will have regained your motivation and developed a realistic action plan to continue steadily progressing toward your weight-loss and lifestyle goals. If you are still struggling, consider taking a break for a few weeks (without forgetting everything you have learned) and refocusing when you feel ready.

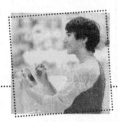

SEVEN

The Busy Person's Maintenance Tips

Losing weight is challenging, but keeping the weight off is even more challenging. With a fast-food restaurant on every corner, jumbo portion sizes, cities so spread out that walking is almost impossible, the dizzying array of cheap and tasty snack items at the grocery store, and the ever-increasing reliance on the Internet for everything from shopping to dating, it's a wonder that anyone is ever able to maintain weight loss. But some do. And obesity researchers and clinicians like me continue to try to figure out why some succeed while many fail.

One group in particular, the National Weight Control Registry, has done extensive work looking at the habits of those who succeed at maintaining their weight loss. This national registry tracks people who have lost weight and kept it off for at least five years. Their findings, as well as those of many others, have helped define many of the traits common to successful weight-loss maintainers. Most of these habits are simply a continuation of the initial weight-loss strategy. Since the NWCR represents a very large and diverse group utilizing varied dieting, exercise, and behavioral strategies, not all of their findings will apply to those who lose weight following my recommendations. But many of their findings are universal and are worth discussing.

In this chapter, I will include many of the NWCR findings as well as those from my own patient experiences. Many of these suggestions will seem obvious or sound familiar. But they should not be ignored or brushed over. For many of you, the real work is just beginning. But don't despair; the longer you maintain, the easier it gets!

DON'T GO "OFF" YOUR PROGRAM

It never ceases to amaze me how people work so hard to lose weight through diet and exercise, only to return to their old habits almost overnight the minute that they reach their goal weight. Just because you have successfully lost weight does not mean that you no longer have to watch your weight. I have yet to see someone become "naturally" thin and eat whatever he or she wants after successful weight loss. The key is to begin your weight-loss program with the intention of building a lifestyle that allows you to enjoy life *and* keep your weight under control. This does not mean that during maintenance you have to watch everything that goes into your mouth for the rest of your life, but you should not have been doing that in the first place.

During weight maintenance, you have somewhat more flexibility in terms of portions and occasional indulgences, but this varies considerably from person to person. The key is to find the right balance for you. You may choose to add one or two starches per day and perhaps one or two fats, but don't change your fundamental approach to eating. Keep eating protein regularly. Research shows that eating slightly more protein can help you successfully maintain weight loss.[1] And don't start skipping meals, especially breakfast. The majority of successful maintainers in the NWCR eat breakfast regularly.[2]

WEIGH YOURSELF REGULARLY

Most obesity experts agree that this is absolutely essential for maintaining weight loss. How often you weigh yourself depends on your confidence in your ability to maintain your weight. For the first few months, I recommend weighing yourself every two weeks. After that, you can weigh at least monthly or anytime your clothes start feeling a tiny bit snug. But just weighing yourself is not enough. You must have a few "call to action" weights. If you gain more than two or three pounds, watch your portions closely for a week or two, or you may want to consider journaling again for a week to see where you may be overdoing it. If your weight goes up by more than five or ten pounds, you must find a way to get back on track or at the very least stabilize your weight as soon as possible. Go back to the basics if you cannot figure out why your weight is creeping back up. Enlist the help or support of a friend, family member, or professional (trainer, doctor, dietitian). Remember that you weigh a lot less than when you started this process, and you may simply need less food (or more exercise) to maintain your smaller physique.

Expand Your Exercise and Activity Options

Findings from the NWCR suggest that most successful weight-loss maintainers exercise at least one hour daily.[3] But if you are a busy person, odds are that you do *not* have this much time per day to devote to exercise. Does that mean that you are destined to fail? Absolutely not. In my experience, the secret to success is to continue exercising as much and in as many different ways as possible and to focus on maintaining an active lifestyle. Take up vigorous hobbies. Experiment with a new exercise class. Go on an active vacation. Sign up for a 5K run or cancer walk. Adopt a dog, or offer to walk your neighbor's dog or a local shelter dog. The key is to exercise *consistently*, and one of the best ways to be consistent is to constantly introduce new activities to prevent boredom. If you are a creature of habit, try to spice up your workouts any way you can. Walk faster or take a different route a few days per week. Do everything you can to stay engaged in your exercise program.

BE CONSISTENT

Research shows that most successful dieters stay relatively consistent in their eating patterns over weekends, holidays, and even vacations.[4] Just as overeating during these times can sabotage your weight-loss efforts, it can interfere with maintenance too, sometimes permanently. Many of my patients have told me about past weight-loss experiences during which one terrible eating weekend or decadent vacation sent them into an eating frenzy from which they could not recover. I'm not suggesting that you never eat another Christmas cookie or drink another margarita on the beach; I'm simply suggesting that you never "turn off" your nutrition knowledge and eat whatever you want in unlimited quantities for an entire weekend, holiday, or vacation. Continue to make the choices that got you this far in the first place. Go ahead and drink that margarita every once in a while, but skip the chips. Eat the Christmas cookie (or three), but skip the eggnog. Have a decadent brunch—followed by a light lunch. Learning to adopt a controlled, flexible approach will keep you healthy for years to come.

DON'T DITCH VEGGIES

Vegetables, as a group, have the fewest number of calories per serving (lowest energy density) in addition to being a great source of filling fiber and cancer-fighting phytonutrients. If you keep your vegetable intake high, while maintaining food intake about the same or even slightly higher, your total caloric intake will stay lower without requiring you to watch your diet as closely. This is one of the keys to maintaining weight loss: built-in calorie control. Don't stop eating veggies and dip when you get home from work famished. Don't quit ordering a salad or vegetable-based appetizer when you go out. Keep experimenting with quick and easy veggie recipes to ensure that you never get bored. If you only do one thing when you reach your goal weight, keep up your vegetable intake and you will increase your chances of maintaining your hard-earned weight loss.

DE-STRESS REGULARLY

Studies have proven that people who have better stress management techniques are much better at maintaining weight loss.[5] Stress and emotional eating are two of the quickest ways to fall back into your old eating patterns and regain weight. It is absolutely essential that you find an outlet other than food for dealing with stress and painful emotions. Many people find meditation helpful. I don't have the patience for regular meditation, but I find exercise to be very beneficial. Not only do you burn calories, but the endorphins produced during exercise help elevate mood and sweat off stress (figuratively, not literally).

Another option, which may be more challenging for busy people, is to minimize stress in any way possible. People who struggle with their weight are often "pleasers," who are more concerned with making sure everyone else is happy than with their own well-being. It is critical that you be somewhat selfish for the sake of stress reduction and maintaining weight loss. Don't stay late at work again if it means grabbing junk food from the vending machine or ordering pizza. Insist that your husband keeps an eye on the kids while you exercise. Skip lunch with your best friend if her recent promotion is going to depress you. Manage stress and you will probably manage your weight as well.

Do "Sweat" the Small Stuff

While small changes can add up to big weight loss, they can add up to slow and steady weight gain as well. After you have lost weight, you need fewer calories because there is less of you than when you began trying to lose weight. Even if you lost weight slowly, ate plenty of lean protein, and did resistance training on a regular basis, you still need less food to maintain your weight than when you were heavier. And even if you do as I suggest and continue eating all the healthy food that you ate while losing weight, you will gain weight if you eat more of it. Keep paying attention to your eating. This does not mean that you have to watch every bite that goes into your mouth, but do pay attention to portion sizes. You can always start with a smaller portion and see how you feel. If you are still hungry, eat more. The food is not going anywhere (unless you got it from a lunch truck!). If you have been very active, have a bit more. Not so active, a bit less. Going out for dinner, cut back a bit on lunch. Just be aware of the little things, and your weight won't creep back up little by little.

If you still believe that weight maintenance is not

challenging, read on and see how one of my most intelli-
gent patients, a surgeon, managed to regain all the weight
he worked so hard to lose by not following my tips.

● ● ●

GA is a surgeon who was referred to me for weight loss. His
goal was to lose twenty pounds and get off all of his blood
pressure medications. He stayed in very good shape for his
job, which often required long hours, standing in the oper-
ating room. He ran five miles several times a week and was
an avid squash player. While his diet was not unhealthy, he
often went long hours without eating and noticed that his
energy level was just not what it used to be.

At our initial meeting, I explained to him the importance
of eating protein-based meals and snacks more regularly
throughout the day to optimize his energy and keep his
blood sugar stable. I suggested that he increase his postrun
breakfast to fuel his body throughout the day. He began
making himself a "power smoothie" with fat-free milk, whey
protein powder, bananas, and peanut butter. This combination really improved his energy level during long, challenging operations. For lunch he opted for the hospital salad bar,
with whatever lean protein was available, and for snacks he
stuck with protein bars and fruit. At night, his wife agreed
to prepare starch for herself only, and he stuck with protein
and vegetables, with an occasional dessert.

After one month, he was down eight pounds, and I suggested that he incorporate resistance training to maintain
or improve his lean body mass. He hired a personal trainer to

design a challenging routine, and after another month he was down six more pounds and was feeling strong and energetic. Over the next month, despite an ankle injury that limited his exercise, he lost another five pounds, and his blood pressure was perfect. At this point, one pound away from his original goal, he decided to try to lose at least ten more pounds, since the first nineteen had been relatively painless.

Over the holidays, he maintained his weight despite frequent parties and extensive travel. After battling a few injuries over the next few months, he managed to lose another five pounds and seemed on track to hit his second goal weight. Then a few things happened that threw him completely off track. He became incredibly busy at work, and several health issues caused him to rethink his eating approach, despite losing twenty-four pounds with the Busy Person's approach. He decided to switch to a very low-fat, vegetarian diet, and I did not see him again for several months.

He came back three months later, up nineteen pounds, frustrated, and ready to once again adopt my nutrition approach. He felt sluggish all the time on a higher-carb diet, despite choosing the highest quality carbohydrates available. I explained that he more than likely had metabolic syndrome and was therefore especially sensitive to both the quality and quantity of carbohydrates in his diet.

He is back on the right track and slowly losing weight again. His story is a great example of how important it is to stick with the basics of this eating approach for good. Even the most successful people you know probably struggle with the same issues you do, but they never give up, and you shouldn't either.

● ● ●

Now that you have finished reading *The Busy Person's Guide to Permanent Weight Loss*, I hope you feel confident that you finally have the tools necessary for simple yet effective weight loss, even with your busy lifestyle. I realize that most people who read this book have struggled with their weight for years, and many have tried every diet plan out there. I understand that it's a bit of a "leap of faith" to truly believe that this diet can and will work for you. All I can say is that over the years I have seen thousands of patients just like you who have tried and failed (or had short-term success) at almost every diet. They came to me with varying levels of faith—most had a healthy amount of skepticism. But those who truly took the time to listen and read the things that I presented to them were surprised to learn how easy permanent weight loss can be.

I hope you will be inspired by the patients from all walks of life presented in this book. Most of them began their weight-loss journey with the same thoughts and beliefs that you may have. Maybe they believed their lifestyle was not compatible with healthy eating due to travel or social obligations. Or they felt they could not stick with the necessary exercise outlined in many popular weight-loss plans or government recommendations. Perhaps they "knew everything" about healthy eating but just could not seem to implement the right eating strategies in their jam-packed schedules. Whatever their reasons for not succeeding in the past, they all slowly adopted many of the suggestions presented in this book and finally found the key to the weight-loss success for which they had spent so much time and energy looking.

I know it won't always be easy for you. Let's face it: nothing in life that is truly worthwhile is always easy. But I know that if you put your mind to it and go through the steps outlined in this book, beginning with goal setting right through maintenance strategies, you can and will be successful at weight loss. And who knows? Maybe I'll be using *you* as an inspiring testimonial for my next book!

APPENDIX A: Protein Bar Chart

GENERAL RECOMMENDATIONS
- Less than 3.5 grams saturated fat is preferable.
- Sugar-to-protein ratio should be approximately 1:1 or less (less sugar than protein if possible).
- The fewer the trans fats the better. A company may list trans fats as zero if there are less than 0.5 g.

Bar	Calories	Fat	Saturated Fat	Carbs	Fiber	Sugar	Protein	Trans Fats?	Exchanges	Notes
Atkins Advantage	220 cal.	11g	7g	25g	11g	0g	17g	No	1 S 2P 1F	Much higher saturated fat
Avid bars	240 cal.	6 g	1.5g	22g	1g	8g	24g	No	1.5 S 3P	Slightly higher calorie bar; women start with $^1/_2$ for snack
Balance	200 cal.	6g	3.5g	23g	0g	18g	14g	Yes	1.5 S 2P	This bar is $^1/_3$ sugar.
Balance Gold	210 cal.	7g	4g	23g	0g	12g	15g	Yes	1.5 S 2P	OK nutrition. Tastes like a candy bar!
Belly Bar	180 cal.	4.5g	1.5g	26g	2g	11g	8g	No	1.5 S 1P	Great for losing the baby weight; all natural, so safe even if you are breastfeeding!
Clif Bar	250 cal.	6g	2g	42g	5g	20g	11g	No	2.5 S 1P	Good for before and/or during long workouts!
Dr. Melina Bar	160 cal.	5g	1.5g	22g	5g	10g	14g	No	1 S 2 P	I designed this bar to taste great and help you lose weight.
EAS AdvantEdge – Carb control	210 cal.	5g	3g	19g	2g	1g	26g	No	1 S 3.5 P	Not great tasting, but healthy; too high in protein for smaller, less active women
GeniSoy Low Carb Crunch	150 cal.	4.5g	3 g	19g	2g	1g	15g	No	1 S 2 P	Great taste; perfect for snacks
Kingbert Healthy Break	175 cal.	5g	<1g	29g	6g	13g	9g	No	1.5 S 1P .5 F	Only all natural bar! Super healthy.
Luna	180 cal.	4.5g	3g	24g	2g	12g	10g	Yes	1.5 S 1.5 P	Slightly less protein; good flavor choices and taste
NuGo	180 cal.	3g	1.5g	26g	2.5g	13g	11g	No	1.5 S 1.5 P	Low glycemic index; very good taste
Power Bar Nut Naturals	210 cal.	10g	1g	19g	3g	8g	10g	No	1.5 S 1 P 1 F	New natural protein bar by Power Bar; good for snacks; higher fat is due to nuts, so it is healthy fat
Pria Complete Nutrition Bar	170 cal.	5g	3.5g	22g	5g	8g	11g	No	1 S 1.5 P	Great tasting (especially choc mint) and good nutrient profile
Smart Zone Crunchy, Hershey's	210 cal.	7g	3.5g	23g	2g	19g	14g	No	1.5 S 2 P	Taste great; low glycemic index; created by Dr. Barry Sears
South Beach Diet Meal Bar	220 cal.	7g	3g	26g	5g	<1g	19g	No	1.5 S 2.5 P	Peanut butter is very good; slightly higher in protein; could work for a meal replacement in a pinch
SlimFast High Protein	200 cal.	7g	2.5g	21g	2g	8g	15g	Yes	1.5 S 2 P	Better than the other SlimFast products. Taste is pretty good.
Think Thin!	240 cal.	10g	4.5g	21g	>1g	0g	20g	No	1.5 S 3 P	Great taste and good nutrition!
Zone Perfect	200 cal.	7g	4.5g	21g	>1g	14g	15g	Yes	1.5 S 2 P	Higher sugar/ok protein; fair choice

* Many low carb bars contain sugar alcohols that count as carbs but not as sugar because they do not have the same effect on the blood sugar as regular sugar. If eaten in excess, they may cause some gastrointestinal side effects.

NOTE: The information presented in this chart may have changed since the publication of this book.

Melina B. Jampolis © 2003

APPENDIX B

Five Ingredients (or Less) Recipes

Remember that cooking is *not* my area of expertise. So the following are a few quick and easy recipes that I have come up with or modified, along with some great ideas from my patients. None of these recipes requires more than five ingredients, because if you are reading this book, you probably don't have time for more than that. Most of the recipes serve two, so double the recipes if you are cooking for the whole family, or save half for lunch the next day. I have included mainly vegetable-based options, since these are the foods that busy people tend to eat less frequently. Also, most of these recipes use precooked products, but feel free to use fresh ingredients if you prefer. When using canned or frozen foods, try to choose lower-sodium options whenever possible. For more ideas, or if you like to cook (and have the time), I suggest getting a lower-fat, healthy carbohydrate cookbook like *The South Beach Diet Cookbook*.

BREAKFAST RECIPES

Fast Frittata for One
In microwave-safe bowl mix:
½ cup cooked fresh or frozen veggies (spinach, peppers, mushrooms)
½ cup egg substitute
Cover and heat in microwave for 1 minute. Stir and heat for
    additional minute.
Optional: Top with 1–2 tablespoons fresh Parmesan, feta, or
    goat cheese.

Quick and Tasty Quiche Cups (bake over the weekend, and reheat
and eat all week)
In a bowl mix:
2 cups cooked spinach (fresh or frozen) or any other
    vegetable (mushrooms, onions, peppers)
1 ½ cups egg substitute
½ cup shredded, reduced-fat cheese, feta, or goat cheese
Pour into muffin tin sprayed with cooking spray (foil muffin
    cups optional).
Bake 20 minutes at 350 degrees.
Makes 6

Apple "Danish" (great for breakfast or a healthy dessert)
On low-carb tortilla, put:
½ thinly sliced apple or ½ cup low-sugar apple sauce
½ ounce–1 ounce part-skim mozzarella cheese or ¼ cup
    low-fat ricotta cheese
Top with cinnamon and Splenda or sugar.
Heat for 20–30 seconds and serve.

DRESSINGS

An easy way to ensure that your dressing covers the entire salad
is to put all the ingredients in a large piece of Tupperware, cover,
and shake for a few seconds.

Dijon Delight Dressing
1 tablespoon Dijon mustard
2 tablespoons plain fat-free yogurt
2 tablespoons balsamic vinegar
Mix well.
Optional: Add 1–2 teaspoons of olive oil and a dash of garlic
powder, or try lemon juice in place of yogurt.

Blue Cheese Dressing
2 tablespoons balsamic vinegar
2 teaspoons olive oil
1-2 tablespoons blue cheese
Mix well.
Salt and pepper to taste (great on pear and walnut salad).

QUICK GOURMET HOT AND COLD SALADS
(ALL RECIPES = 2 SERVINGS)

Easy Appetizer Salad
Mix:
1 bag of lettuce
1 cup cherry tomatoes
1 ounce of crumbled goat cheese
Top with 2 tablespoons of rice vinegar (usually found in the
gourmet or Asian food section).
Optional: Add 1–2 tablespoons chopped walnuts (if you have not
had too much fat for the day).

Tasty Two-Bean Salad
Combine and toss:
2 cups cooked green beans
2 tablespoons crumbled feta
¼ to ½ cup chickpeas
2 teaspoons olive oil
2 tablespoons vinegar
Optional: Add 3–6 ounces chopped chicken, salmon, or tuna.

Savory Salmon Salad
Combine:
½ can cannellini beans (rinsed and drained)
1 6-ounce can of salmon
2 tablespoons vinegar
2 tablespoons crumbled feta
Serve over 2–3 cups of lettuce.

Chicken Salad
Mix:
1 can chicken
2 tablespoons rice vinegar
2 teaspoons olive oil
2 tablespoons crumbled blue cheese
Optional: Add ½ cup grapes.
Serve over mixed greens.

Gourmet Vegetable Salad
Combine:
1 bag of mixed veggies (fresh or cooked in microwave)
1 jar or can of artichoke hearts
2–3 teaspoons olive oil
½ teaspoon garlic (optional)
Top with 2 tablespoons fresh Parmesan cheese.
Optional: Add 3-6 ounces chopped chicken, salmon, or tuna for a
    complete meal.

Asian Chicken Slaw Salad
Mix:
2 cups coleslaw mix
1 large can chicken
¼ cup honey-roasted nuts
2 tablespoons low-fat vinaigrette dressing or 1 tablespoon
    low-sodium soy sauce and 2 teaspoons sesame oil

Tasty "Taco" Salad
Top 2–3 cups of lettuce with:
½ can chicken

½ cup cherry tomatoes
½ cup black or pinto beans
1–2 tablespoons premade guacamole
Use salsa for dressing.

Nice and Easy Nicoise Salad
Top 2–3 cups Bibb lettuce (or any lettuce you prefer) with:
1 can tuna or two 3-ounce tuna fillets
½ cup green beans
1 egg (cut into fourths)
Drizzle with Dijon mustard-based dressing.
Optional: Top with 1–2 tablespoon capers.

Go Greek Salad
Combine:
1 sliced cucumber
1 cup chopped tomato
½ chopped red onion
¼ cup reduced-fat feta cheese (regular is OK too)
¼ cup red wine vinegar
If you don't want to slice the vegetables, go to your favorite salad bar and get them precut. Combine with reduced-fat feta cheese and vinegar at home.

Ten Quick and Tasty Vegetable "Recipes"

You can always simply sauté vegetables in olive oil and garlic or top them with a tasty premade sauce or one to two tablespoons of freshly grated Parmesan for added flavor, but here are a few more ideas to get you and your family more excited about vegetables.

- Heat bag of frozen cauliflower in microwave until soft; mash with a fork and add 1 tablespoon light butter spread or 2 teaspoons olive oil and ½ teaspoon chopped garlic.
- Heat fresh or frozen green beans, spray with I Can't Believe It's Not Butter Spray or 2 teaspoons olive oil, and toss with 2 tablespoons of slivered almonds.

- Sauté prebagged fresh or frozen spinach with 2 teaspoons olive oil, ½ teaspoon garlic, and mushrooms.
- Combine 1 tablespoon olive oil, 1 teaspoon lemon juice, and ½ teaspoon garlic. Toss with 1–2 cups steamed broccoli or asparagus.
- Heat 1 tablespoon peanut butter and ½ cup reduced-sodium chicken broth in microwave and pour over cooked vegetables (optional: add chicken for easy meal).
- Mix bag baby carrots with 2 tablespoons honey, 2 tablespoons light margarine, and 1 tablespoon lemon juice. Cover and heat in microwave for 6 minutes.
- Heat 2 cups fresh or frozen Brussels sprouts and toss with 1 ½ tablespoons syrup and 2–4 teaspoons of butter. Add salt and pepper to taste.
- Slice eggplant, brush with olive oil, and broil for a few minutes on each side. Sprinkle with fresh Parmesan.
- Combine 1–2 tablespoons olive oil, 1 teaspoon cumin, ½ teaspoon curry, and salt and pepper to taste. Toss with 2 cups cooked broccoli and cauliflower.
- Sauté or heat 2 cups cooked spinach in 2 teaspoons of olive oil and 1 teaspoon garlic. Stir in 2 tablespoons feta cheese. Salt and pepper to taste. Optional: Add ½ cup chopped tomato or cooked lentils.

Quick Main Course Ideas

Easy Chicken Chili
In a pot or bowl combine:
1 can chicken
½ can kidney or black beans
1 large can chopped tomatoes
1 can tomato paste (optional)
1 packet chili seasoning (or season with chili powder, cumin, and cinnamon to taste)

Heat in microwave or on stove until warm, and serve alone, or
pour over 2 cups of broccoli, one of my favorite things to do.

Easy Mexican Wrap
In a large sauté pan or bowl, combine:
1 can chicken
½ can fat-free refried beans or black beans
1 jar salsa
Heat on stove or in microwave until warm.
Spoon into one or two low-carb tortillas and eat.
Optional: Top with 1–2 tablespoons guacamole.

2-Minute Tortilla Soup
In a pot or bowl, combine:
½ of a 12-ounce jar of salsa
1 large can cooked chicken or 1 ½ cups of cooked chicken strips
1 ½ cups low-sodium chicken broth
½ can of drained beans (optional)
Heat in microwave or on stovetop until warm.
Makes 2 servings.

Tasty Stir-Fry
In a pot or bowl, combine:
½ cup reduced-sodium chicken broth
1 tablespoon reduced-sodium soy salt
1 large can drained chicken, heated in a skillet for 2 minutes (add
    spices for flavor)
2 cups cooked fresh or frozen broccoli (heat in microwave to cook)
Heat in microwave or on stovetop until warm.
Optional: Add 1 teaspoon garlic if you like, or use vegetable broth
    and fresh or frozen shrimp in place of chicken.

APPENDIX C

Frequently Asked Questions

If I lower starch intake below my recommended servings per day or cut them completely, will I lose weight more quickly?

The answer for most people, especially men, is probably yes. Some of my patients like to jump-start their diets by cutting starches from all meals except breakfast. They do generally lose weight more quickly, but they also lose a considerable amount of water weight and often a small amount of calorie-burning muscle mass as well. The rapid weight loss does not continue for long, and most people quickly become bored with the limited food choices and slowly add starches back into their diet at the recommended levels. Women seem to have a more difficult time cutting starches completely out of their diet and often report depression and fatigue if they try to cut starches too drastically.

Another approach if you want to speed up your weight loss would be to cut bread, pasta, and rice from your diet initially, and eat only the highest quality starchy carbohydrates, like high-fiber cereal, beans, and sweet potatoes. Many patients lose weight slightly faster when limiting themselves to these types of starches. But the majority of my patients, especially those who are super-busy and on the run constantly, find it almost impossible to remove bread completely from their diets. By balancing out their day correctly and making the best choices possible, they often end up losing just as much weight, if not more, in the long run.

What is BMI? Should I focus on this number instead of weight?

BMI (body mass index) is a ratio of your height to your weight. A BMI of below 25 is normal; 25–29 = overweight; and greater than 30 = obese. The medical community uses BMI as a measure of obesity in research and general practice. The problem with this measurement is that it does not distinguish between lean body mass (muscle, water, bone) and fat mass. For example, a muscular woman could have a BMI in the overweight range if she has an extra ten pounds of lean body mass. I find it much more useful to look at body fat percent, but not everyone has access to this type of testing. Many of the inexpensive body fat scales work fairly well if used at the same time each day, though it is important to understand that in the morning, when you are dehydrated, the body fat percent will be slightly overestimated with these types of scales. Men should aim for a body fat percent below 20, and women should aim for a body fat percent of 25 if they are premenopausal and 30 percent if they are peri- or postmeno-pausal. It is important for women to realize that female-specific body fat, such as breast tissue, will impact your goal fat percent. Women with a smaller bust size feel more comfortable with less than 25 percent body fat, while women with a larger bust size may find it challenging to get below 25 percent body fat. A nutrition or fitness professional can help you more accurately define your body fat goals.

I don't seem to be successful at weight loss without some accountability. Any suggestions?

This is a very common issue. Most of my patients feel they need to see me regularly to stay on track even when they know exactly what they need to do. You have a couple of options to deal with this issue. One solution would be to find a weight-loss buddy with whom you check in on a regular basis. I'm also a big fan of Weight Watchers, and while my recommendations may not be exactly in line with theirs, I think the group support, regular weigh-ins, and camaraderie at their meetings are terrific and can be very beneficial for someone who enjoys group settings.

I noticed that many convenience foods are higher in salt. If I have high blood pressure, is it still OK to eat them?

The government recommends a maximum of 2,400 mg of sodium (salt) per day. Many frozen and prepackaged foods do contain a large amount of sodium, so in general, it is always best to choose lower-sodium options. However, the impact of weight loss on lowering blood pressure in most people is much more important than the effect of lowering sodium, so if you need to eat a bit more prepackaged (and portion-controlled) food to lose weight, it is probably safe. It is also just as important to eat enough potassium each day to keep blood pressure down. Fruits and vegetables are the best sources of potassium, so you have another reason to make sure you eat more of them daily.

What exactly are sugar alcohols? Are they safe?

Sugar alcohols, including sorbitol, mannitol, xylitol, erythritol, lactilol, and maltilol are commercially produced sweeteners that offer several advantages over sugar. They have a much lower glycemic index; do not cause cavities; and because they are not absorbed completely by the body, they have fewer calories per gram than regular sugar, so they can be helpful for weight control. Due to the fact that they are not fully absorbed by the body, excess consumption can lead to gas and diarrhea. However, all of these sweeteners are considered safe for dietary use in moderate amounts. [1]

What about artificial sweeteners?

Artificial sweeteners, including saccharin, aspartame, acesulfame K, and sucralose are considered food additives and have essentially no calories. All are considered safe even at very high doses. Some health experts recommend against these types of sweeteners, but there is little evidence that they have negative health effects.[2] For weight loss, if the average American consuming 95 grams of sugar per day replaced those added sugars in their diet with artificial sweeteners, they would save 380 calories per day. In my opinion, as with many things, the potential beneficial impact on weight loss outweighs any theoretical objections that health experts may have to artificial sweeteners. As with all of my recommendations, I suggest consuming artificial sweeteners in moderation.

Is it OK for convenience to use meal replacements instead of meals or snacks?

Absolutely, as long as you eat high-quality meals too. In fact, research shows that portion-controlled entrees and meal- and snack-replacement bars can help with both weight loss and maintenance.[3, 4] The benefits are obvious: built-in portion control, minimal planning, and convenience. But it is not a good idea to replace all of your meals with meal replacements. Not only will you more than likely be deficient in some vitamin or nutrient, but you will also miss out on the pleasure of eating. If you do choose meal replacements, studies show that bars tend to be more filling than shakes, so if you are someone who gets hungrier more often, you may want to stick with protein bars (see Appendix A).

Is it bad to eat almost the same thing every day?

That depends on what you are eating every day. Many of my patients seem to do better when they stick to a routine during the week and get a bit more variety on weekends. As long as you are focusing on the basic nutrition principles and eating enough fruits and vegetables, you are probably OK. In fact, research shows that people with less variety in their diet seem to do better with weight loss and maintenance.[5] One of my most successful patients used to chart out his meals for the week every Sunday night. He rotated through the same meals over and over, and yet he never seemed to get bored. He deviated occasionally during the holidays and for things like poker night with the boys or dinner at the French Laundry, one of the most famous restaurants in the country. He lost forty-six pounds in six months and now has the cholesterol and physique of a thirty-year-old (in his mid-fifties).

My trainer said I should exercise first thing in the morning on an empty stomach. Is this true?

To my knowledge there has never been any conclusive research showing that exercising on an empty stomach has any real benefit for weight loss. Even if you burn a bit more fat this way, you will probably be so hungry by the time you eat that you will consume more than you would have if you had eaten something before exercise. In addition, if your energy is lower from not eating, your workout will probably not be as vigorous and you will burn fewer calories. I tell my patients to try to get at least a little breakfast, even if it is only an apple, half a protein bar, or a slice of whole-grain bread and a tablespoon of peanut butter on the way to the gym.

Since metabolism is so important, do I have to get it checked to lose weight?

Not necessarily. Most people assume that a slow metabolism is the cause for their inability to lose weight. I perform metabolism testing on most of my patients, and slow metabolism is rarely to blame. The only time I have seen patients with a slow metabolism is if they have untreated thyroid disease, have lost a lot of muscle mass due to an injury or inactivity, or are training for an endurance sports event and undereating significantly. The most important thing you can do is have your doctor make sure that your thyroid is normal. If you are interested in having your metabolism tested, many gyms and weight-loss centers now offer this sort of testing. I use a device made by Korr Medical (www.korr.com), and many gyms have a device made by HealtheTech.

Should I eat differently if I have thyroid disease?

Maybe. Some evidence suggests that eating too much soy protein blocks both the absorption and action of thyroid medication. If you are taking thyroid medication, I recommend that you eat soy protein in moderation, and you may want to avoid it around the time of day that you take your thyroid medication (which should be taken at least thirty minutes before meals). I saw a patient who was on thyroid medication and was not losing weight for months despite following all of my recommendations. After thoroughly analyzing her diet, I realized that she was eating soy protein bars in the morning, a few hours after taking her thyroid medication. I suggested that she cut the bars for a few weeks to see what happened. Within a week she felt much more energetic and began losing weight. It is not necessary to cut soy protein completely, but you may want to cut back if you eat large amounts (for example, vegetarians). It is also important not to take thyroid medication with calcium, antacids, or iron supplements, as they will interfere with the absorption.

Is coffee OK? What about diet soda?

I'm not sure why or when coffee became taboo for dieters. Research shows that coffee may actually decrease your chances of getting type 2 diabetes.[6] In addition, coffee is no longer felt to be a risk factor for high blood pressure,[7] and national recommendations by the Joint National Committee on Prevention, Detection, Evaluation, and Treatment of High Blood Pressure (JNC 7) no longer supports restriction of coffee or caffeinated beverages for the treatment of high blood pressure. The bigger issue with coffee and weight loss is not the coffee itself but what you put in it. A large soy latte may seem harmless, but at 270 calories, it can interfere with weight loss. And at 500 calories, that large whole-milk mocha with whipped cream can do some real damage to your diet. Having one every day can add up to a one-pound weight gain, or prevent a one-pound weight loss, each week!

Diet soda is a bit more controversial due to the artificial sweeteners and chemicals, but there is little research showing any negative health or weight loss effects, so I do not require that patients cut out diet soda unless they feel like it is affecting their weight loss.

I'm a vegetarian. Any tips?

Depending on what type of vegetarian you are, this program may be a bit more challenging. If you eat fish, dairy, and eggs, you will have no problem finding numerous lean-protein choices for meals and snacks. If you don't eat fish, I suggest that you take a fish oil supplement, as it is very difficult to get adequate amounts of omega-3 fatty acids exclusively from plant sources. If you don't eat dairy, make sure to take a calcium and vitamin D supplement. You may find getting protein at breakfast and snacks tricky. Consider buying protein powder to make smoothies or add to oatmeal. If you are a total vegan and don't eat any fish, dairy, or eggs, it will be tougher, but not impossible, to follow my recommendations. Regular and low-fat tofu is an excellent source of protein, as is protein powder. Beans and nuts are good sources of protein, but beans are very high in carbohydrates, and both beans and nuts are high in calories. If you have metabolic syndrome or high normal blood sugar, following a vegan diet will make losing weight much more complicated. You will probably have to exercise significantly more to be successful.

My doctor told me I have high cholesterol. Are they any natural ways of lowering cholesterol?

This is one of my favorite questions. The ability of a healthy diet, regular exercise, and a few key supplements to lower cholesterol surprises even my most open-minded medical colleagues. An incredible research study a few years ago compared what the researchers thought was the perfect heart-healthy diet with the average dose of a powerful cholesterol-lowering medication. After only one month, both groups had a 30-percent reduction in bad cholesterol.[8]

I realize that the perfect diet is difficult to follow in the real world every day, but even incorporating more heart-healthy foods on a regular basis can have huge effects on cholesterol reduction. In addition, I recommend fish oil supplements to all of my patients with high cholesterol to lower triglycerides and raise good cholesterol. I have also seen very good results lowering total and bad cholesterol with a concentrated green tea extract. The following box lists the heart-healthy foods used in the research study I mentioned, along with a few others. Try to regularly incorporate as many as you can into your diet.

SUPER HEART-HEALTHY FOODS

enriched margarines (Benecol)

soy protein (milk, burgers, etc.)

almonds

oatmeal

barley

psyllium (Metamucil)

cruciferous vegetables (okra, eggplant, broccoli, Brussels sprouts, cauliflower)

apples

blueberries

salmon

whole or ground flaxseeds

I always see the heart-rate training poster in the gym. Should I be paying attention to this or wearing a heart-rate monitor?

The cardiovascular conditioning and fat-burning zones listed on the posters in the gym are too generic to really be useful, and from a weight-loss standpoint, they do not matter. Here's why: If you exercise at higher intensities (higher heart rate), you will burn a higher percentage of calories from carbohydrates than fats but more total calories. If you work at lower heart-rate zones, you will burn a higher percent of calories from fat but fewer total calories. The goal for weight loss is to burn more calories. You can do this by exercising more intensely (at a higher heart rate) or for a longer period of time at a lower intensity. People with less time are better off exercising at higher heart rates for shorter periods of time. If you are the type of person who likes to follow numbers, by all means wear a heart-rate monitor. But it is in no way necessary for weight loss.

I thought I was not supposed to eat after dinner. Is that true?

I'm not quite sure where this idea came from, but my suggestion is that if you are hungry after dinner, eat. It is probably not a great idea to go to bed very hungry, as this may interfere with sleep, which can cause weight gain. To my knowledge, there is no science that proves that calories consumed after 7 PM are more likely to be stored as fat. Research does suggest that eating a higher percent of your total daily calories at night is associated with obesity.[9] To avoid this, try to spread calories evenly throughout the day rather than piling them on at night. But there is no need to restrict calories completely at night. I recommend, of course, that you eat a protein-based snack such as yogurt and fruit, or peanut butter and half an apple.

I have gout—should I worry about eating more protein?

Yes and no. While the true effect of dietary protein on gout is slightly controversial, diets higher in animal protein, including chicken, meat, and fish, can increase gout attacks. On the other hand, recent research shows that diets higher in dairy and soy proteins can actually decrease gout attacks.[10] Increasing water intake and decreasing alcohol intake will also help, and it is important to not cut carbohydrates too much, as they can help prevent gout attacks. Finally, weight loss will probably help the most, so the best thing to do is follow my general recommendations for weight loss, which are centered on a balanced diet.

APPENDIX D

Shopping Lists

While I am not a big fan of processed food, I admit that I probably could not manage easily without it. In a perfect world we would all make our own soups and yogurt and eat only organic meats, fruits, and vegetables. In the real world, many of my patients simply don't have the time or budget to eat perfectly and must rely on premade, packaged foods. Following are examples of products that I personally like and many that my patients have recommended to me. This list is certainly not comprehensive, so I urge you to experiment with things not on the list. Just make sure to compare labels and make the best choices possible. Also, to keep your salt intake under control, try to limit yourself to one course of processed food per meal. For example, try not to eat a high-salt soup with a high-salt frozen dinner. Start with raw vegetables and dip instead. Or start with the soup, and then have a stir-fry instead of a frozen dinner. The fresh foods will balance out the salt in the more processed foods.

Food Staples

Items to buy regularly no matter where you shop

- ❑ Eggs (for breakfast or hard-boiled for snacks)—one dozen (egg substitute is OK too)
- ❑ Lean protein (low-fat deli slices, canned chicken or tuna, cooked or frozen chicken and turkey breasts, frozen fish and shrimp)
- ❑ Low-sugar, low-fat yogurt (for breakfast, snacks, dessert)—buy at least seven
- ❑ Low-fat cottage cheese (for breakfast or snacks)
- ❑ High-fiber cereal (add to yogurt or eat for breakfast)—aim for a minimum of 5 grams of fiber per serving
- ❑ Frozen vegetables—get a variety of several bags for easy dinners
- ❑ Premade sauces—perfect for quick and tasty vegetable or lean-protein topping
- ❑ Fresh and frozen fruit—fresh and portable fruits for snacks, frozen fruit to defrost for breakfast or desserts
- ❑ Precut vegetables and tasty low-fat dips—perfect for appetizers and snacks
- ❑ Low-carbohydrate tortillas—trust me, these are incredible and you can wrap almost anything in them and they taste great
- ❑ Dijon mustard (for quick dip or dressing)
- ❑ Oil (olive, canola) and vinegar
- ❑ Nuts (buy in individual servings or pour ¼ cup into Baggie)
- ❑ Canned beans (refried or regular, any kind you like for quick and easy salads and toppings)
- ❑ Salsa—great for easy recipes; healthy topping and easy salad dressing
- ❑ Cooking spray—for those who cook, a must-have for stir-fries, omelets, and more
- ❑ Low-fat salad dressing—better tasting than fat free and research has shown that a little fat may be better for nutrient absorption in vegetables
- ❑ Reduced-salt chicken broth (for quick soup or sauté)
- ❑ Reduced-salt soy sauce (for quick sauté or dressing)

General Grocery Items

Some of these items may be hard to find in large chain grocery stores; you may have better luck in natural or specialty food stores. You do not have to limit yourself only to items on this list. Just use it to get started in the right direction.

S = starch   P = protein oz.   F = fat   V = vegetable
Fr = fruit   D = Dairy

Protein and Dairy
DiGiorno shredded Parmesan cheese: 2 tablespoons = ½ P ½ F
   (put 1–2 tablespoon on veggies for flavor)
Athenos crumbled feta cheese: 2 tablespoons = ½ P ½ F
   (put 1–2 tablespoons in salads for flavor)
Alouette Light Garlic and Herb Cheese Spread: 2 tablespoons =
   ⅓ P ½ F
Boursin Light cheese spread: approx. 2 tablespoons = ½ P ½ F
String cheese: 1 P ½ F
Laughing Cow Light Garlic & Cheese Wedge: 1 = ½ P ½ F
   (I love this spread on low-carb tortillas)
Jarlsberg Light Swiss: 1 slice = 1 P ½ F
   (presliced, so built-in portion control)
Mini Babybel Light Cheese: 1 round = 1 P
   (built-in portion control)
Foster Farms roasted chicken strips: 3 oz. = 3 P
   (great for quick stir-fries, or toss on salads)
Tyson Fajita Chicken Breast Strips (precooked): 3 oz. = 3 P
   (perfect rolled up in a low-carb tortilla with salsa)
Starkist Tuna Fillets: 5 oz. (full packet) = 6 P
   (easy heat-and-eat lunch or dinner)
Starkist Chunk White Tuna packet in water: 1 = 3 P
   (great for on-the-go lunch)
Chicken of the Sea Salmon pouch: 1 = 2 P (easy on-the-go omega-3s)
Bumblebee albacore tuna easy can: 1 = 3 P
Canned chicken (Swanson, Valley Fresh*, Hormel): 2 oz = 2 P
   (* lowest salt)

Lightlife Smart Ground Taco and Burrito Meatless Crumbles:
⅓ cup = 1 ½ P (Mix with salsa and fat-free refried beans, and
you will not be able to tell that this is not meat!)
Papa Cantella's Gourmet Poultry Sausages, Smoked Chicken &
Turkey Pesto: 1 link = 3 P ½ F (lower fat than most brands)
Knudsen's On-the-Go Cottage Cheese (low-fat or nonfat):
1 serving = 2 P (great on-the-go option)
Fage's 0 percent or 2 percent Total Greek Yogurt: 1 cup = 2 P
(+ 1 F for 2 percent) This is one of my favorite products!
Yoplait Light Smoothie: 1 bottle = 1 D
Dannon Light 'n Fit Carb & Sugar Control Smoothie: 1 bottle = 1 D
Designer Protein Whey Powder French Vanilla or Chocolate:
1 scoop = 2 ½ P (great for smoothies or add to oatmeal)

Sauces, Dressings, and Spreads
Smucker's low-sugar jam: 1 tablespoon = 25 calories
(skip the sugar free; tastes very artificial)
Knott's Berry Farm light: 1 tablespoon = 20 calories
Take Control or Benecol light spread: 1 tablespoon = 1 F
(contains heart-healthy plant sterols)
Smart Balance light spread: 1 tablespoon = 1 F
(contains heart-healthy omega-3s)
Marukan rice vinegar: 1 tablespoon = 0 calories
(great as easy salad dressing)
Heinz Chili Sauce: 1 tablespoon = free
Kraft Mesquite BBQ Sauce: ¼ cup = 1 V ½ S
Annie's Naturals Roasted Red Pepper Vinaigrette:
1 ½ tablespoon = 1 F
Annie's Naturals Raspberry Vinaigrette (low fat): 2 tablespoons = ½ F
Girard's Light Champagne dressing: 2 tablespoons = 1 F
Newman's Own Lighten Up Low-Fat Sesame Ginger Dressing:
2 tablespoons = ½ F
Newman's Own Light Balsamic Vinaigrette: 2 tablespoons = 1 F
Spectrum Light Canola Mayo: 1 tablespoon = ½ F
(If you really love mayonnaise, go for this healthy version.)
McCormick or Lawry's seasoning mixes: chili, burrito, taco
(slightly high in salt but quick and easy flavor)

Emeril's Roasted Pepper pasta sauce: ½ cup = ½ F 1 V
Amy's Low Sodium Organic Pasta Sauce: ½ cup = 1 V
Francis Coppola Organic Arrabbiata Spicy Pasta Sauce:
    ½ cup = ½ F 1 V
Classico Fire Roasted Tomato & Garlic Pasta Sauce: ½ cup = 1 V

Bread, Cereals, Other Starches (high fiber is key)

Oroweat whole-grain rye bread: 1 slice = 1 S (3 g. fiber)
Oroweat whole-grain nut English muffin: 1 = 2 S (5 g. fiber)
Sara Lee Heart Healthy Plus: 1 slice = 1 S (4 g. fiber)
Milton's whole grain: 1 slice = 1 S (5 g. fiber)
Food for Life Ezekiel Bread: 1 slice = 1 S
Sara Lee whole wheat pita: ½ = 1 S (2 g. fiber)—great for pita
    pocket sandwiches
La Tortilla Factory Whole Wheat Low Carb Tortillas:
    1 tortilla = ½ S (8 g. fiber; I eat several of these every day
    in place of bread.)
Mission Carb Balance tortilla: 1 = 1 S (8 g. fiber—great for wraps,
    burritos, and more)
Quaker Take Heart Instant Oatmeal: 1 packet = 2 S
    (6 g. fiber—super heart healthy)
Quaker regular oatmeal, instant: 1 packet = 1 S (3 g. fiber)—
    add Splenda and cinnamon for flavor
Quaker Weight Control Oatmeal, Cinnamon: 1 packet = 1 ½ S 1 P
    (6 g. fiber)
Kashi instant oatmeal: 1 packet = 1 ½ S 1 P (5 g. fiber)
Kashi GoLean cereal: 1 cup = 1 ½ S 1 ½ P (10 g. fiber)
Kashi GoLean Crunch! cereal: 1 cup = 2 S 1 P
    (8 g. fiber; ¼ to ½ cup tastes amazing in yogurt)
Fiber One Honey Clusters: 1 ¼ cup = 2 S (14 g. fiber)
Weight Watchers Flakes 'n Fiber Cereal: ½ cup = 1 S 1 P (6 g. fiber)
All-Bran Buds: ⅓ cup = less than 1 S (13 g. fiber—great way to add
    crunch and fiber to yogurt)
Barbara's Puffins cereal: ⅔ cup = 1 S (6 g. fiber, taste great, good
    for kids too)
Health Valley Organic Fiber 7 Multigrain Flakes: 1 cup = 2 S
    (7 g. fiber)

Nature's Path Organic Pumpkin FlaxPlus Granola: ½ cup = 1 S 1 F
Nature's Path Optimum Power Breakfast, Flax/Soy/Blueberry
  (cereal): 1 cup = 2 S 1 P (10 g. fiber)

Snacks and Crackers
Kellogg's All-Bran Bars, Brown Sugar Cinnamon: 1 = 1 ½ S (5 g.
  fiber—great for on-the-go breakfasts)
Kashi Trail Mix Chewy Granola bar: 1 bar = 1 S 1 F ½ P
South Beach Diet High Protein Cereal Bar: 1 = 1 S 1 P
  (3 g. fiber—easy snack option)
GeniSoy Soy Crisps: 17 crisps (3.5 servings/container) = ½ S 1 P
  (great instead of chips)
Quaker Soy Crisps BBQ flavor: 18 crisps = 1 P ½ S
GeniSoy Soy Nuts: ¼ cup = 1 ½ P ⅓ S (great as a snack with fruit)
Triscuits, reduced fat: 5 = 1 S (2 g. fiber)
Ak-Mak crackers: 3 ½ crackers = 1 S (2.5 g. fiber)
Kashi Tasty Little Crackers (TLC): 10 crackers = 1 S
Doctor Kracker Flatbread: 1 flatbread = 1 S (these whole-grain,
  organic crackers taste terrific)
South Beach Diet Snack Crackers, Whole Wheat: 1 = 1 S (3 g. fiber;
  individually packaged, so instant portion control)

Soups and More (choose lower-salt when possible)
Rosarita 98-percent fat-free refried beans: ½ cup = 1 S 1 P
  (great for quick and healthy burritos)
Rosarita low-fat black refried beans: ½ cup = 1 S 1 P
Vegetarian chili, canned (Dennison's, Hormel, Stagg, MorningStar
  Farms, Lightlife): 1 cup = 2 S 1 ½ P (11 g. fiber—more energy
  dense, so watch serving size)
Westbrae Natural Organic Lentils or Chili Beans: ½ cup = 1 S 1 P
  (lower in salt)
S&W Black Beans or Kidney Beans, 50-percent-less sodium:
  ½ cup = ½ S 1 P
Simply Asia Soy Noodle Soup Bowl: 1 = 1 P ½ S (just add water,
  easy on-the-go snack or starter)
Imagine organic soups (in a box): 1 cup; also lower in salt, so
  larger servings are OK

Creamy Butternut Squash: 3 V

Creamy Potato Leek: 2 V ½ S

Amy's organic soups: 1 cup serving; lowest in salt, so may have
larger serving if desired

Low Fat Black Bean Vegetable: 1 ⅓ S 1 P

Chili: 1 ⅓ S 1 P ½ F

Minestrone: ½ S 2 V

Progresso soups: 1 cup serving; high in sodium, so limit serving
size to 1 cup

Minestrone: 1 ½ V ½ S

Vegetable: 3 V

Lentil: 1 S 1 P

Chicken Noodle: ½ S 1 P

Beef Barley Vegetable: ½ S 1 V 1 P

Campbell's: 1 cup serving; all flavors are similar to Progresso for
exchanges although slightly lower in salt than Progresso but
still high, so limit serving

Select Mexican Style Chicken Tortilla: 1 S 1 P

Select New England Clam Chowder, 98-percent Fat-Free: 1 S 1 P

Select Italian Tomato with Basil & Garlic, Gold label: 3 V

Select Golden Butternut Squash, Gold label: 3 V

Select Blended Red Pepper Black Bean: ½ S 2 V

Chunky Grilled Chicken & Sausage Gumbo: 1 S 1 P

Soup at Hand, Blended Vegetable Medley: 3 V
(easy on-the-go option)

Healthy Request Cream of Mushroom, reduced sodium:
½ cup = 2 V (add water)

Frozen Foods
(choose lower-salt, whole-grain options whenever possible)
MorningStar Farms sausage link: 2 = 1 ½ P (great for breakfast)
Lightlife Smart Bacon (soy based): 2 strips = 1 P
Lean Pockets breakfast: 1 = 1 S 1 P ½ F
Kashi GoLean Waffles (plain or blueberry): 1 waffle = 1 S
(3 g. fiber; top with berries or low-sugar jam and cottage
cheese instead of syrup)
Van's 97-percent Fat-Free Waffles: 1 waffle = 1 S (2.5 g. fiber)

Birds Eye Voila! Roasted Garlic Chicken & Vegetables:
1 cup cooked (2.5 per bag) = 1 ½ P 2 V
Contessa Chicken Stir-Fry: 1 ¾ cups (3 per bag) = 2 P 3 V
(higher in salt, so watch the number of servings)
Lean Cuisine Carb Conscious frozen entrees: read individual
labels to figure out food exchanges
Weight Watchers Smart Ones Chicken Marsala = 3 P 2 V
Healthy Choice no-starch options: read individual labels to
figure out food exchanges
Cedarlane Garden Vegetable Enchiladas: 1 (2/container) = 1 P 1 S 1 V
Gordon's grilled frozen fish filets: 1 = 2 P
(quick and easy dinner protein)
Lean Pockets Reduced Fat Meatballs & Mozzarella: 1 = 3 P 1 S
(easy on-the-go lunch)
Digiorno Harvest Wheat frozen pizza: ⅕ pizza = 2 S 2 P (4 g. fiber)
Amy's Brown Rice & Vegetables Bowl (made with tofu):
1= 2 S 1 P 1 V (good lunch option)
MorningStar Farms Cheddar Burger (vegetarian): 1 = 2 P ½ S
MorningStar Farms Philly Cheese Steak Burger (vegetarian):
1 = 1 ½ P ½ F
Boca Burger (vegetarian): 1 = 2 P
MorningStar Farms Tomato & Basil Pizza Burger (meatless):
1 burger = 1 ½ P ½ F ½ S

Healthy Dessert Options and Miscellaneous:
Sugar-free popsicle: 1 = free food (great dessert)
Breyers No Sugar Added Frozen Fruit bar: 1 = ½ F
Weight Watchers desserts = varied nutrition; most count as 1–2
starches. Good for portion control
Almondina biscuits: 4 biscuits = 1 ½ S ½ F (low sugar, all natural)
Droste Pastilles Extra Dark (chocolate pieces):
2 pieces = ½ F ⅓ S (good for portion control)
Jell-O, Sugar Free = free food
Jell-O Pudding, Sugar Free Fat Free = 1 D
Hansen's Diet Soda

APPENDIX E: Food Journal

Date: ___ / ___ / ___ Mon Tues Wed Thu Fri Sat Sun

Breakfast: Time _____

_____

Starch ❑ ❑ ❑ Protein ❑ ❑ ❑ ❑ Fat ❑ ❑ ❑ Fruit ❑ ❑ ❑
Vegetable ❑ ❑ ❑ Dairy ❑ ❑

Morning Snack: Time _____

_____

Starch ❑ ❑ Protein ❑ ❑ Fat ❑ ❑ Vegetable ❑ ❑ Dairy ❑ ❑

Lunch: Time _____

_____

Starch ❑ ❑ ❑ Protein ❑ ❑ ❑ ❑ ❑ ❑ Fat ❑ ❑ ❑ Fruit ❑ ❑ ❑
Vegetable ❑ ❑ ❑ Dairy ❑ ❑

Afternoon Snack: Time _____

_____

Starch ❑ ❑ Protein ❑ ❑ Fat ❑ ❑ Vegetable ❑ ❑ Dairy ❑ ❑

Dinner: Time _____

_____

Starch ❑ ❑ ❑ Protein ❑ ❑ ❑ ❑ ❑ ❑ ❑ Fat ❑ ❑ ❑ Fruit ❑ ❑ ❑
Vegetable ❑ ❑ ❑ Dairy ❑ ❑

Evening Snack: Time _____

_____

Starch ❑ ❑ Protein ❑ ❑ Fat ❑ ❑ Vegetable ❑ ❑ Dairy ❑ ❑

TOTALS:
Starch _____ Protein _____ Fat _____ Fruit _____ Vegetable _____ Dairy _____

Water: ❑ ❑ ❑ ❑ ❑ ❑ ❑ ❑ ❑ ❑ ❑ Daily Vitamins: ❑

Exercise:
Cardio: (type, duration) _____

Strength: (body parts worked) _____

Other: _____

Weekly Worksheet

Date: _____ to _____

List at least one thing that you did well this week in all three categories.
(Example: Ate regularly, walked 3 times, planned weekend meals)

Nutrition:

1. _____

2. _____

3. _____

Exercise:

1. _____

2. _____

3. _____

Behavior:

1. _____

2. _____

3. _____

List at least one thing that you would like to work on in all three categories.
(Example: Eat more vegetables, increase amount of weights, stop negative thinking)

Nutrition:

1. _____

2. _____

3. _____

Exercise:

1. _____

2. _____

3. _____

Behavior:

1. _____

2. _____

3. _____

List at least one short-term goal.
(Example: Fit into smaller pants in six weeks, jog one mile without stopping)

1. _____

2. _____

3. _____

NOTES

ONE: The Busy Person's Basic Principles

1. Carol S. Johnston, Carol S. Day, and Pamela D. Swan, "Postprandial Thermogenesis Is Increased 100% on a High-Protein, Low-Fat Diet Versus a High-Carbohydrate, Low-Fat Diet in Healthy, Young Women," *Journal of the American College of Nutrition* 21, no. 1 (February 2002), 55–61.
2. M. P. St. Onge, F. Rubiano, W. F. Denino, A. Jones Jr., D. Greenfield, P. W. Ferguson, S. Akrabawi, and S. B. Heymsfield, "Added Thermogenic and Satiety Effects of a Mixed Nutrient vs. a Sugar-Only Beverage," *International Journal of Obesity* 28 (2004), 248–253.
3. D. Layman, E. Evans, J. Baum, D. Erickson, and R. Boileau, "Dietary Protein and Exercise Have Additive Effects on Body Composition During Weight Loss in Adult Women," *Journal of Nutrition* 135 (2005), 1903–10.
4. G. R. Hunger, J. P. McCarthy, M. M. Bamman, "Effects of Resistance Training on Older Adults," *Sports Medicine* 34(5) (2004), 329–48.
5. D. S. Weigle, P. A. Breen, C. C. Matthys, H. S. Callahan, K. E. Meeuws, V. R. Burden, J. Q. Purnell, "A high-protein diet induces sustained reductions in appetite, ad libitum caloric intake, and body weight despite compensatory changes in diurnal plasma leptin and ghrelin concentrations," *American Journal of Clinical Nutrition* 82 (2005), 41–8.
6. M. P. Lejeune, E. M. Kovacs, and M. S. Westerterp-Plantenga, "Additional Protein Intake Limits Weight Regain After Weight Loss in Humans," *British Journal of Nutrition* 93, no. 2 (February 2005), 281–9.
7. S. Iwao, K. Mori, and Y. Sato, "Effects of Meal Frequency on Body Composition During Weight Control in Boxers," *Scandinavian Journal of Medicine and Science in Sports* 6, no. 5 (1996), 265–72.
8. Yunsheng Ma, Elizabeth R. Bertone, Edward J. Stanek III, George W. Reed, James R. Hebert, Nancy L. Cohen, Philip A. Merriam, and Ira S. Ockene, "Association Between Eating Patterns and Obesity in a Free-Living US Adult Population," *American Journal of Epidemiology* 158, no. 1 (2003), 85–92.
9. J. S. Garrow, M. Durrant, S. Blaza, D. Wilkins, P. Royston, and S. Sunkin, "The Effect of Meal Frequency and Protein Concentration on the Composition of the Weight Lost by Obese Subjects," *British Journal of Nutrition* 45, no. 1 (1981), 5–15.
10. H. R. Farshchi, M. A. Taylor, and I. A. Macdonald, "Decreased Thermic Effect of Food After an Irregular Compared with a Regular Meal Pattern in Healthy Lean Women," *International Journal of Obesity* 28, no. 5 (March 2004), 653–60.
11. Mark Pereira, Janis Swain, Allison Goldfine, Nader Rifai, and David Ludwig, "Effects of a Low-Glycemic Load Diet on Resting Energy Expenditure and Heart Disease Risk Factors During Weight Loss," *Journal of the American Medical Association* 292, no. 20 (November 24, 2004), 2482–90.
12. Jennie Brand-Miller, Thomas M. S. Wolever, Kaye Foster-Powell, and Stephen Colagiuri, *The New Glucose Revolution: The Authoritative Guide to the Glycemic Index—the Dietary Solution for Lifelong Health* (New York: Marlowe & Company, 2003).
13. C. Maffeis, S. Provera, L. Fillipi, et al, "Distribution of Food as a Risk Factor for Childhood Obesity," *International Journal of Obesity and Related Metabolic Disorders* 24 (2000), 75–80.

14. Brian Wansink, James E. Painter, and Jill North, "Bottomless Bowls: Why Visual Cues of Portion Size May Influence Intake," *Obesity Research* 13 (2005), 93–100.
15. Nicole Dilberti, Peter L. Bordi, Martha T. Conklin, Liane S. Roe, and Barbara J. Rolls, "Increased Portion Size Leads to Increased Energy Intake in a Restaurant Meal," *Obesity Research* 12 (2004), 562–8.
16. T. V. Kral, L. S. Roe, and B. J. Rolls, "Combined Effects of Energy Density and Portion Size on Energy Intake in Women," *American Journal of Clinical Nutrition* 79, no. 6 (June 2004), 962–8.
17. Barbara Rolls, *The Volumetrics Eating Plan* (New York: HarperCollins Publishers, 2005).
18. M. J. Lamonte, S. N. Blair, "Physical Activity, Cardiorespiratory Fitness and Adiposity: Contributions to Disease Risk," *Current Opinion in Clinical Nutrition and Metabolic Care* 9(5) (2006 September), 540–6.

TWO: The Busy Person's Guide Customized for You

1. C. Johnston, "Strategies for Healthy Weight Loss: From Vitamin C to the Glycemic Response," *Journal of the American College of Nutrition* 24, no. 3 (2005), 158–165.
2. Yong-Woo Park, Shankuan Zhu, Latha Palaniappan, Stanley Heshka, Mercedes R. Carnethon, Steven B. Heymsfield, "The Metabolic Syndrome: Prevalence and Associated Risk Factor Findings in the US Population from the Third National Health and Nutrition Examination Survey, 1988–1994," *Archives of Internal Medicine* 163 (2003), 427–36.
3. Marc-Andre Cornier, W. Troy Donahoo, Rocio Pereira, Inga Gurevich, Richard Westergren, Sven Enerback, Peter J. Eckel, et al, "Insulin Sensitivity Determines the Effectiveness of Dietary Macronutrient Composition on Weight Loss in Obese Women," *Obesity Research* 13 (2005), 703–9.
4. Michael B. Zemel, Warren Thompson, Anita Milstead, Kristin Morris, and Peter Campbell, "Calcium and Dairy Acceleration of Weight and Fat Loss During Energy Restriction in Obese Adults," *Obesity Research* 12 (2004), 582–9.
5. Rozemarijn Vliegenthart, S. Oei Hok-Hay, Annette P. M. van den Elzen, Frank J. A. van Rooij, Albert Hofman, Matthijs Oudkerk, and Jacqueline C. M. Witteman, "Alcohol Consumption and Coronary Calcification in a General Population," *Archives of Internal Medicine* 164, no. 21 (November 22, 2004), 2355–60.
6. H. A. Raynor, R. W. Jeffery, D. F. Tate, R. R. Wing, "Relationship Between Changes in Food Group Variety, Dietary Intake, and Weight During Obesity Treatment," *International Journal of Obesity Related Metabolic Disorders* 28(6) (2004 June), 813–20.
7. "Making Green Vegetables Taste Good," Tufts University Health & Nutrition Letter, July 2004, 6.
8. Maggie B. Covington, "Omega-3 Fatty Acids," *American Family Physician* 70, no. 1 (July 1, 2004), 133–40.

THREE: The Busy Person's Meal Ideas

1. Holly R. Wyatt, Gary K. Grunwald, Cecelia L. Mosca, Mary L. Klem, Rena R. Wing, and James O. Hill, "Long-Term Weight Loss and Breakfast in Subjects in the National Weight Control Registry," *Obesity Research* 10, vol. 2 (February 2002), 78–82.
2. H. R. Farshshi, M. A. Taylor, and I. A. Macdonald, "Deleterious Effects of Omitting Breakfast on Insulin Sensitivity and Fasting Lipid Profiles in Healthy Lean Women," *American Journal of Clinical Nutrition* 81, no. 2 (2005), 388–96.
3. Jillon S. Vander Wal, Jorene M. Marth, Pramod Khosla, Catherine Jen, and Nikhil V. Dhurandhar, "Short-Term Effects of Eggs on Satiety in Overweight and Obese Subjects," *Journal of the American College of Nutrition* 24, no. 6 (2005), 510–15.
4. M. C. Nachtigal, Ruth E. Patterson, Kayla L. Stratton, Lizbeth A. Adams, Ann L. Shattuck, and Emily White, "Dietary Supplements and Weight Control in a Middle-Age Population," *Journal of Alternative and Complementary Medicine* 11, no. 5 (October 2005), 909–15.

5. David J. Maron, Guo Ping Lu, Nai Sheng Cai, Zong Gui Wu, Yue Hua Li, Hui Chen, Jian Qui Zhu, Xue Juan Jin, Bert C. Wouters, and Jian Zhao, "Cholesterol-Lowering Effect of a Theaflavin-Enriched Green Tea Extract," *Archives of Internal Medicine* 163 (June 2003), 1448–53.

6. A. Khan, M. Safdar, M. M. Ali Khan, K. N. Khattak, R. Z. Anderson, "Cinnamon Improves Glucose and Lipids of People with Type 2 Diabetes," *Diabetes Care* 26(12) (2003 December), 3215-8.

7. Michael Boschmann, Jochen Steiniger, Uta Hille, Jens Tank, Frauke Adams, Arya Sharma, Susanne Klaus, Friedrich Luft, and Jens Jordan, "Water-Induced Thermogenesis," *Journal of Clinical Endocrinology & Metabolism* 88, no. 12 (December 2003), 6015–19.

8. S. A. French, M. Story, R. W. Jeffery, "Environmental Influences of Eating and Physical Activity," *Annual Review of Public Health* 22 (2001), 309–35.

FOUR: The Busy Person's Exercise Strategies
1. Lorraine Lanningham-Foster, Lana J. Nysse, and James A. Levine, "Labor Saved, Calories Lost: The Energetic Impact of Domestic Labor-Saving Devices," *Obesity Research* 11, no. 10 (October 2003), 1178–81.

2. Timothy J. Quinn, Jenny R. Klooster, and Robert W. Kenefick, "Two Short, Daily Activity Bouts vs. One Long Bout: Are Health and Fitness Improvements Similar Over Twelve and Twenty-Four Weeks?" *Journal of Strength and Conditioning Research* 20, vol. 1 (February 2006), 130–35.

3. G. R. Hunger, J. P. McCarthy, M. M. Bamman, "Effects of Resistance Training on Older Adults," *Sports Medicine* 34(5) (2004), 329–48.

FIVE: The Busy Person's Behavior Tips
1. B. Wansink, J. Painter, "Proximity's Influence on Estimated and Actual Candy Consumptions," North American Association for the Study of Obesity 2005 Annual Scientific Meeting Abstract.

SIX: The Busy Person's Real-World Challenges
1. Pamela S. Haines, Mary Y. Hama, David K. Guilkey, and Barry M. Popkin, "Weekend Eating in the United States Is Linked with Greater Energy, Fat, and Alcohol Intake," *Obesity Research* 11, no. 8 (August 2003), 945–49.

2. Ibid.

3. S. B. Roberts and J. Mayer, "Holiday Weight Gain: Fact or Fiction?" *Nutrition Review* 58, no. 12 (December 2000), 378–9.

4. P. A. Mole, "Impact of Energy Intake and Exercise on Resting Metabolic Rate," *Sports Medicine* 10(2) (1990 August), 72–87.

5. M. Tanofsky-Kraff, S. Z. Ynovski, "Eating Disorder or Disordered Eating? Non-normative Eating Patterns in Obese Individuals," *Obesity Research* 12(9) (2004 September), 1361–6.

SEVEN: The Busy Person's Maintenance Tips
1. M. P. Lejeune, E. M. Kovacs, and M. S. Westerterp-Plantenga, "Additional Protein Intake Limits Weight Regain After Weight Loss in Humans," *British Journal of Nutrition* 93, no. 2 (February 2005), 281–9.

2. Holly R. Wyatt, Gary K. Grunwald, Cecelia L. Mosca, Mary L. Klem, Rena R. Wing, and James O. Hill, "Long-Term Weight Loss and Breakfast in Subjects in the National Weight Control Registry," *Obesity Research* 10, vol. 2 (February 2002), 78–82.

3. Ibid.

4. Rena R. Wing and Suzanne Phelan, "Long-Term Weight Loss Maintenance," *American Journal of Clinical Nutrition* 82, no. 1 (July 2005), 222S–225S.
5. K. Elfhag and S. Rossner, "Who Succeeds in Maintaining Weight Loss? A Conceptual Review of Factors Associated with Weight Loss Maintenance and Weight Regain," *Obesity Review* 6, vol. 1 (February 2005), 67–85.

APPENDIX C: Frequently Asked Questions

1. "Position of the American Dietetic Association: Use of Nutritive and Nonnutritive Sweeteners," *Journal of the American Dietetic Association* (2004), 255–75.
2. Ibid.
3. Sandra M. Hannum, LeaAnn Carson, Ellen M. Evans, Kirstie A. Canene, E. Lauren Petr, Linh Bui, and John W. Erdman Jr, "Use of Portion-Controlled Entrees Enhances Weight Loss in Women," *Obesity Research* 12, no. 3 (March 2004), 538–48.
4. K. C. Haddock, W. S. Poston, P. Pace, R. Reeves, M. M. Pinkston, and J. P. Foreyt, "Weight Loss with Meal Replacements and Meal Replacement Plus Snacks: The Results of a 24-Week Randomized Trial," North American Association for the Study of Obesity 2004 Annual Scientific Meeting Abstract.
5. H. A. Raynor, R. W. Jeffery, S. Phelan, J. O. Hill, R. R. Wing, "Amount of Food Group Variety Consumed in the Diet and Long-Term Weight Loss Maintenance," *Obesity Research* 13(5) (2005 May), 883–90.
6. Rob M. Van Dam, Walter C. Willet, JoAnn C. Manson, and Frank B. Hu, "Coffee, Caffeine, and the Risk of Type 2 Diabetes: A Prospective Cohort Study in Younger and Middle-Aged US Women," *Diabetes Care* 29 (February 2006), 398–403.
7. Wolfgang C. Winkelmayer, Meir J. Stampfer, Walter C. Willet, and Gary C. Curhan, "Habitual Caffeine Intake and the Risk of Hypertension in Women," *Journal of the American Medical Association* 294, no. 18 (November 9, 2005), 2330–35.
8. David J. A. Jenkins, Cyril W. C. Kendall, Dorothea A. Faulkner, Tri Nguyen, Thomas Kemp, Augustine Marchie, Julia M. W. Wong, et al, "Assessment of the Longer-Term Effects of Dietary Portfolio of Cholesterol-Lowering Foods in Hypercholesterolemia," *American Journal of Clinical Nutrition* 83, no. 3 (March 2006), 582–91.
9. C. Maffeis, S. Provera, L. Fillipi, "Distribution of Food as a Risk Factor for Childhood Obesity," *International Journal of Obesity Related Metabolic Disorders* 24 (2000), 75–80.
10. Hyon K. Choi, Karen Atkinson, Elizabeth W. Karlson, Walter Willet, and Gary Curhan, "Meat, Seafood, and Too Little Dairy Are Risk Factors for Gout," from "Purine-Rich Foods, Dairy and Protein Intake, and the Risk of Gout in Men," *New England Journal of Medicine* 350, no. 11 (March 11, 2004), 1093–1103.

ABOUT THE AUTHOR

Melina Jampolis, M.D., is a board-certified internist and physician nutrition specialist (one of only two hundred in the country). She specializes exclusively in nutrition for weight loss and disease prevention and treatment. A graduate of Tufts University and Tufts School of Medicine, she completed her residency in internal medicine at Santa Clara Valley Medical Center, a Stanford University teaching hospital.

In 2005, Dr. Jampolis hosted a ten-episode diet program called *FitTV's Diet Doctor* on the Discovery Network's FitTV. She currently serves on the advisory board and contributes regularly to a women's lifestyle and wellness digital interactive magazine, *VIVmag* (www.vivmag.com). She also lectures throughout the country on nutrition for weight loss and wellness and continues to see patients in private practice with offices located in San Francisco and Burlingame.